Stronger Than The Storm

One Woman's Journey of Adventure, Adversity and Unbreakable Spirit

Dear Gemma,
I hope you enjoy it!
Felicity
x

Felicity Ashley

Dear Hannah,

I hope you enjoy it!

Felicity
x

**Stronger Than The Storm
One Woman's Journey of Adventure,
Adversity and Unbreakable Spirit**
Copyright © Felicity Ashley 2025

The right of Felicity Ashley to be identified as the author of this work has been asserted by her in accordance with the Copyright, Designs and Patents Act, 1988.

All rights reserved. No part of this book may be reproduced, stored in a retrieval system or transmitted in any form or by any means (electronic, mechanical, photocopy, recording, scanning or other) except for brief quotations in critical reviews or articles, without the prior written permission of the publisher.

ISBN: 9781068489105 Paperback

Published by: Inspired By Publishing

For Mum and Dad, for showing me how to live life.

For Paul, for your unwavering love and support.

For Sam, Ben and Grace, for giving me my "why."

Acknowledgements

Nobody achieves anything significant alone. We surround ourselves with people who can support us through the hard times and lift us higher in the good times. I call these people my "support crew."

Some are there for the long haul, while others come and go more fleetingly, playing a part when the time is right.

To start at the very beginning, I want to thank Mum and Dad. My parents have been a wonderful and enduring influence on my life, from nature to nurture. They are my role models for living life with authenticity, compassion, kindness, generosity of spirit, faith, hope and love. They gave me my foundations by instilling in me the self-belief to try anything and the encouragement to find my path in life. They've been there through thick and thin – never judging, always loving.

Equally constant through my life are my siblings, James and Pip. Sparring partners through childhood, they helped me find a competitive edge and kept me on my toes. Through adulthood, they've always been there as friends, supporters, advisers, encouragers, confidants and people with whom to share the highs and lows.

Pip, thank you for asking me to row an ocean with you. It speaks volumes that you'd want to do it with your sister, someone who, during our teenage years, you would rather have fed to sharks, I'm sure. I'm honoured and grateful to have shared such an incredible experience with you. Getting to know you on a different level and seeing your strength and humour was one of the greatest privileges of our adventure. Your advice, which convinced me to say "yes," will stay with me for life.

Family can be overwhelming, so to those who have become part of my family – my brother-in-law David, my sister-in law Sally and their reams of offspring – thank you for throwing yourselves into our family with humour and grace. You've created such a bustling, chaotic, happy band of brothers, sisters and cousins, upholding the family values that have always been core to my existence.

I want to give a particular shout-out to David for planting the seed for the Atlantic row and inspiring me to do it. His selfless and heartfelt enthusiasm and support for our row were infectious, keeping any flickering doubt at bay.

And of course, front and centre of my world is Paul – the person who willingly (and sometimes unwittingly) supports everything I do. He's given me three wonderful children, and I'm so grateful. Thank you, Paul. You haven't just supported me through the rollercoaster of recent life, but you've thrown yourself into every challenge it has posed for you, taking on responsibility that many would have shied away from. For better or worse, for richer or poorer, in sickness and in health – you are there by my side, even when we were oceans apart. Thank you for upholding your side of the marriage bargain so graciously, and for challenging me. If Carlsberg did husbands and fathers…

Sam, Ben and Grace, thank you for giving me my "why." For being the brilliant, brave, funny and lovable people you are, and for being the reason I do most things in life. You've taught me so much about myself, the good and the sometimes not-so-good. Thank you for playing your part in my adventures. You are my reason to row an ocean, my reason to come home safely, my light at the end of the tunnel through cancer treatment, my joy in the everyday. You didn't have a choice in the journey but chose to navigate it with courage, enthusiasm, support and love. "Don't be rubbish, Mummy," is very sound advice. I'm immensely proud of you all.

To Chris and Barry, Paul's parents, thank you for welcoming me into your family and instilling in Paul the values that make him the brilliant husband and father he is. I'm sure it can't have been easy for you to watch your son's wife and mother of your grandchildren disappear across the Atlantic on a crazy adventure, but you took it all in your stride, and have shown me nothing but support, love and encouragement. Thank you for being there to pick up the pieces when our lives have been swept off course, and for your incredible influence.

"If you want to go fast, go alone. If you want to go far, go together." This proverb rings true in so many ways when it comes to rowing an ocean. While some people choose to row an ocean solo, I feel so blessed to have shared the experience with Jo, Lebby and Pip. Thank you, all of you, for being a dream team. Thank you for putting your trust and confidence in me, and for sharing and bearing, as well as baring, so much. I look back on what we achieved together, and most importantly, how we achieved it, with awe and gratitude. You made the low points endurable and the high points even higher.

Jo and Lebby, thank you for being such a significant part of my life now. Thank you for your stories, camaraderie, determination, spirit and strength during the row and for your love and support through the storms that followed. I sincerely hope there will be another chapter, another adventure for "The Mothership" – ideally, before we become "The Grandmothership."

Jo, Lebby, Pip and I may have been the ones grafting out the 1.5 million oar strokes it took to row an ocean, but many, many people helped us do that. Taking two months out of life as a working mum requires a lot of planning and goodwill, with family, friends and colleagues rallying around to help. Having the support of my employers at Centrica was incredibly important, so a special thank you goes to my manager, Ruth Brougham, and to the CEO, Chris O'Shea, for championing and supporting me. Thank you to everyone who made this possible, from those who gave financial backing and our boat, including Michael, Tom, Tritax and Centrica, to those who supported us technically, including Duncan, Alex and The Atlantic Campaigns team. To the friends, family and colleagues who helped with logistics, and the thousands who cheered us on and helped us raise over £80,000 for our charities – we couldn't have done it without you.

To everyone who has ever shared their personal cancer story or contributed to raising awareness of symptoms, from the bottom of my heart, thank you. I, for one, have benefited beyond measure. The gift of awareness saves lives. Because of people like Ed, Anna and Dame Deborah James, I can look forward to seeing my children grow up, and my family has been spared the heartache that so many families have to endure. I hope that, in my own way, I can pay this forward and help others navigate a difficult journey.

I couldn't write an acknowledgements section without a heartfelt thank you to everyone in the National Health Service (NHS) who contributed to my treatment. I have no doubt there were hundreds in the background whom I didn't meet but who paved the way for my treatment journey and continued surveillance. In particular, I would like to thank the wonderfully kind and pragmatic nurse and consultant who gave me such brilliant advice in the minutes following my diagnosis. Thank you, too, to Kat Baker, my surgeon, for treating me not just as another patient, but as an individual. And lastly, thank you to the oncology team of Professors Anne and David Kerr, who looked after me so brilliantly during chemotherapy and beyond. They're the reason I'm able to share my story.

When one door closes, another one opens. Becoming a speaker (and now author) was not something I ever envisaged. It's a tremendous privilege to have a platform to influence and help people and businesses through my experiences. After leaving my corporate role, I was lucky to have time to explore other avenues and to have people who acted as my sounding boards, giving me advice, guidance or a gentle nudge in the right direction. My coach, Katherine Walker, gave me valuable food for thought, which led to a brain-picking session with adventurer, speaker, author and friend, Paula Reid, and an introduction to the Oracle of the speaking world, Maria Franzoni. A huge thank you to Maria, Mary Tilson-Wharton and Elliot Kay for guiding me through this new world, and thank you to the speaking community for welcoming me with open arms. In particular, thank you to Emma Henderson, my speaker partner-in-crime with whom I've been so lucky to share this journey.

Writing a book can feel like a monumental challenge, and many people – some of whom will not know that they helped me – helped me climb this latest mountain.

Joanne Rose, thank you for planting the seed. I remember our conversation when you said, "There's a book in there."

With a sprinkling of water, light and food from others, the seed grew shoots and roots and blossomed when I was introduced to Matt Bird, whose writing course guided me to a completed manuscript.

For the journey from a manuscript to the book you're reading now, I'd like to give a huge thank you to my publisher, Inspired By Publishing, and my book mentor, Angela Haynes-Ranger, who has held my hand throughout the editing and publishing journey.

Sometimes, we're lucky, and people reach out to offer support. But often, we need to look for the right people to support us and have the courage to ask for help. By asking for help and helping others collectively, we can achieve so much more. Whatever oceans lie before you, having the right support crew around you makes all the difference between pipe dreams and reality, and between surviving or thriving through storms.

Contents

Introduction	1
Chapter 1 - The Formative Years	5
Chapter 2 - The Dodgy Hip	25
Chapter 3 - Feel the Fear and Do It Anyway	39
Chapter 4 - You Don't Have to Be Great to Start, but You Do Have to Start to Be Great	53
Chapter 5 - Hanging in the Balance	75
Chapter 6 - Losing Sight of Land	89
Chapter 7 - Boat Life	101
Chapter 8 - Rowing Through Storms	119
Chapter 9 - The Nightmare Before Christmas	141
Chapter 10 - Ahoy, Land Ahead!	155

Chapter 11 - My Next Challenge Chose Me	173
Chapter 12 - Keep Calm and Carry On	181
Chapter 13 - Why *Not* Me?	195
Chapter 14 - Life Can Be Cruel	211
Chapter 15 - Losing an Anchor	227
Chapter 16 - The Rollercoaster of Chemotherapy	237
Chapter 17 - Finding My Light at the End of the Tunnel	251
Epilogue	259

Introduction

I'm an "ordinary" working mum of three. After a successful but unremarkable journey through school and university, I spent the majority of my career to date in marketing, working my way up the food chain to lead teams for some of the UK's largest organisations.

I experienced the inevitable undulations of business life, including periods of organisational change and job uncertainty, the financial crisis of the late 2000s, the more recent energy crisis and the challenges of working and parenting through the pandemic. I learned about myself, business, people, teamwork and leadership. I learned how to manage change and adversity and achieve ambitious goals. However, none of these gave me any notions of writing a book.

I'd love to say that publishing this book culminates a lifelong dream, a major tick on the bucket list. But it isn't – quite the contrary.

I've said, on many occasions, that I'd rather stick pins in my eyes than write a book. People find this strange since I now spend a good chunk of my working time writing, and I'm in the working world as a professional speaker, where published authors are two-a-penny. (Sometimes, I have to pinch myself when I think about all the incredible and inspirational people surrounding me in my work.) But after years of churning out obligatory essays at school and university, purely to get a decent grade and only to be skim-read by a teacher or lecturer before disappearing into oblivion, I was, frankly, sick to the back teeth of writing.

So, what changed? Life. It gave me a story to tell.

Life has taken me on a rollercoaster ride over the last few years, catapulting me from the euphoria of becoming one of fewer than 250 women to have rowed an ocean to the grim reality of a life-changing health condition.

If I've learned anything through this period, it's that there is nothing as constant as change. The world moves in mysterious ways, taking us on paths we hadn't planned. If we're to flourish, we have to be willing to change with it.

You cannot imagine how you're going to react when you hear the words, "You have cancer." It triggered a compulsion to start talking about my experiences, hoping that sharing my challenges would help others facing something similar.

My journey has given me not only a story and lessons to share but also a purpose, a need and a desire to do so.

When you have sufficient motivation, anything is possible. What started as a few investigatory conversations about professional speaking turned into a 360° career pivot, from corporate marketer to speaker. Alongside finding my feet and voice on the stage, the seeds for this book were planted.

I've surprised myself by how much I've enjoyed the process of writing it. It's been therapeutic and cathartic. There have been genuine tears (of laughter and grief) as I relive my story through the pages.

I don't pretend to be a superhero on a pedestal. I'm an ordinary, working mother of three whose life took extraordinary twists and turns. Some of those paths were ones I chose to take, and others were diversions that forced me to take a different route.

This book is not just about my journey, but also about how I navigated those twists and turns. It's about the many people who have shared the journey, making the highs higher and the lows more bearable. It's about the lessons that I've learned along the way. It's not intended to be a "woe is me" story, but an uplifting tale of the unlikely, and often messy path I've trodden through adversity and beyond. This book will tell you about stubborn determination paired with faith, hope and love.

The lessons are as applicable to the everyday ripples we face in our personal or business worlds as they are to the (hopefully) more occasional oceans and storms that come our way.

Wherever you are in life, and whatever challenges you face now or in the future, I hope my story inspires you to believe you can be your own version of extraordinary. You can cross your own oceans, however big the storms.

Thank you for reading my story.

Chapter 1
The Formative Years

Standing on the finishers' podium of "The World's Toughest Row" in English Harbour, Antigua, alongside my three crewmates, Pip, Jo and Lebby, was a "pinch me" moment. Fewer than 250 women had ever rowed an ocean. We were four of them. This achievement was not the realisation of a lifelong dream or something I'd worked towards for longer than I could remember. This was not something that "people like me" – mid-life, working mums – did. It was for adventurers, extreme sports athletes and otherworldly human beings who were braver, stronger, younger and fitter than I was. Yet here we were, taking our place amongst them, and fitting right in.

At that moment, I realised that ordinary people can do extraordinary things. It is not necessarily talent that separates the extraordinary from the ordinary, but mindset, the right people around you and a capacity and willingness to put in the effort, stroke after stroke, day after day. And that is something that I've always had.

I had a wonderfully happy but unremarkable childhood. My dad was self-employed for most of his career, running a small chain of local newsagents before turning 40 and buying a small Victorian folk museum. Mum was an orthoptist, taking a break from her career to raise their three children and returning to work once my younger sister was in primary school.

I'm the middle child, born in 1976, with an older brother, James, and a little sister, Pip. We were born and bred in rural Wales. While we had a comfortable childhood, it was also a relatively simple one. There were lots of self-made outdoor activities. I spent my time roaming the fields, making mud pies, picking blackberries, and chasing my siblings around with the decapitated neck of a goose. Growing up as one of three children relatively close in age meant competition was part of daily life. Being competitive was thus a characteristic honed from birth. In sibling terms, it was survival: jostling for the best seat on the sofa or control of the TV remote; racing to be first in the bath to avoid the plug end, or, later, the murky waters left behind; arguing over who got stuck in the middle seat of the car, jabbed by elbows on both sides; and sprinting up the stairs to lock yourself in the toilet while your siblings waited, cross-legged, for as long as you could make them.

Having an older brother meant I was always trying to keep up, pushing myself further than I might otherwise have done, and taking risks I would otherwise have avoided. Equally, having a younger sister meant looking over my shoulder, trying to keep one step ahead and in the "natural pecking order" of life.

One summer holiday, when we were on holiday in West Wales, James had ridden off on his bike with a couple of friends, and I was determined not to be left behind. I didn't want to be seen as the little kid by the big boys. I wasn't quite as proficient on two wheels as they were, but I carried on regardless, bumping over the field and track down the hill, grimacing through gritted teeth. I gripped the handlebars so hard my knuckles turned white, becoming increasingly out of control. As I sped faster and faster down the hill, the wind whipping my hair across my face and the tension of impending disaster making every limb rigid, it was all I could do to balance and stay upright. Steering fell by the wayside, and I veered off-road, bouncing over ruts and clumps before careering into a deep pit of stinging nettles, my new bike buried in the vicious foliage. I lay there for a few moments staring at the clouds passing in the sky, eyes blinking back tears of shock, embarrassment and frustration, tentatively moving my head, arms and legs to check for damage.

The smarting of the nettles on my bare arms and legs roused me from my daze, and I picked myself up and clambered out of the pit, every inch of skin angrily throbbing with the sting, dragging my bike behind me.

I spent the rest of the day smothered in calamine lotion, my pride wounded by the little escapade – but not irrevocably so. Although a minor incident, it's something I'll always remember because it revealed so much about who I am: quietly competitive, unwilling to be left behind, and ready to push myself out of my comfort zone to keep up. I don't like being boxed in by gender or age, and I'm someone who willingly steps up to a challenge.

My parents have been a constant influence on and an inspiration to me. The older and wiser I get, the more I recognise and appreciate everything they have given James, Pip and me. We couldn't have asked for a more loving, supportive or grounded start to life.

I cannot think of better role models for marriage. We celebrated their 50th wedding anniversary shortly before Dad died, and I honestly can't remember one single argument. Dad's golden rule was never to go to sleep on an argument; to my knowledge, they never did. It was a marriage deeply rooted in their Christian faith, mutual respect, friendship, partnership and abiding love. That's not to say they didn't occasionally differ in their views. While Dad was remarkably rational and open-minded in most respects, one occasion stands out because it was unfathomably out of character.

During our teenage years, when the Doc Martin craze was at its peak, Mum agreed to take Pip and me to Cardiff to buy a pair of DM boots, using our own hard-earned pocket money. Objectively, Doc Martin boots are very "sensible" footwear for girls, providing ample protection and space for young feet to grow, unlike the pointy-toed, kitten-heeled alternatives. However, Dad had a different opinion. For some reason, Dad railed against the Doc Martin boot craze with an irrational reaction to the innocent boot, which I can only assume hailed from an archaic view of how young ladies should present themselves.

Needless to say, when we arrived home, clomping around in our shiny new cherry-red boots, he did not share our enthusiasm for our investment. We tiptoed around him (metaphorically if not literally), a mixture of pride and nerves spilling over into barely-contained giddiness. He was furious and refused to speak to or even look at either Mum, Pip or me. When we sat down for lunch a little later, I focused only on the food on my plate, not risking looking up and making eye contact for fear of disintegrating into nervous fits of giggles. We sat in uncharacteristic silence, the loud ticking of the clock and clashing of cutlery echoing in the void left by the usual family chatter.

Something had to give, and fortunately, a piglet came to the rescue. As if reflecting the farcical nature of the disagreement, it launched itself through the window alongside the table, landing with a squeal and crash of splintering glass alongside us.

The sudden chaos was too much for Dad's jangled nerves to take, and he abruptly pushed his chair back and marched out, leaving the rest of us to laugh until our sides hurt, shoe the piglet out of the house and clear up the broken glass. This story has become a family legend for its absurdity, finding its way into Dad's eulogy as evidence that even the most upstanding, level-headed and open-minded people have their foibles.

Faith has always guided and influenced us as a family through life, both overtly and subconsciously. As children, Sundays were spent going to Church and Sunday school. Every meal started with the ritual of grace (spoken or sung – the louder, the better). Christmas wouldn't have been Christmas without wrapping up in our thickest layers to withstand the icy chill of a church service before a present could be opened or chocolate consumed.

It wasn't so much the overt practices of being brought up as Christians, but rather the Christian principles and behaviours that shaped my parents – and, I believe, rubbed off on us as children – that served as a guiding light throughout life. We were blessed with a life filled to the brim with unconditional love, kindness, thoughtfulness and respect, where family is central to our existence and time together is something we cherish and look forward to.

My maternal grandfather was ordained a priest after a military career, and my Dad followed suit. On his 70th birthday, he dropped a bombshell and said he would follow an ordination journey. Although it was a surprise, it was entirely consistent with his natural leaning towards helping others. Seeing him respond to his calling and find his purpose later in life filled me with pride and admiration. It was also a powerful lesson in the magnetic force of a purpose to give you the strength, motivation and resilience to overcome any challenges in your path.

I'm asked often whether my love of physical challenges is something I've inherited or learned from my parents, but it isn't. It would be something of a stretch to describe Mum and Dad as sporty. They were always reasonably active (mainly thanks to always having a dog as part of the family and the hands-on work involved in renovating houses), but participating in sports was not something I ever remember them doing. Dad loved his rugby, but was very much an armchair supporter, bellowing advice in his finest Welsh accent, which was reserved only for rugby watching.

The only exception was a short-lived dalliance with running. Having decked themselves out in new trainers and tracksuits, they limbered up on the doorstep and made it as far as one lap around the outside of the house (a small cottage) before abandoning the idea. I'm fairly sure that was the only time Dad wore a pair of trainers. From then on, they remained on a shelf, gathering dust.

Fast-forward a few years, and I think both Mum and Dad were a little bewildered when all three children developed more than a passing interest in sport. I attribute that to the opportunities and encouragement offered to us throughout our school days. Mum and Dad sacrificed a lot to give us a private school education, affording us ample opportunity to enjoy a wide variety of sports.

I relished the sense of community and team spirit that sport offered. I have fond early memories of being on the netball and rounders team in primary school and not-quite-so-fond memories of cold, wet cross-country runs and seemingly endless laps around the athletics track.

Secondary school brought a wider variety of sports. While I never excelled at anything, I always had a go and was passably good at most things. A good all-rounder is a fair description of my school days, whether from an academic or sporting perspective. But an unremarkable achievement didn't come effortlessly, and what I lacked in talent, I made up for in effort. I was a people pleaser. I wanted to do well and was quietly competitive – a survival instinct learned through being the middle child – and I worked *hard*.

Mum recently unearthed some of my old primary school reports. What struck me was the consistency of feedback from my first year right through to leaving for secondary school. "A happy and cooperative little pupil who should do well in school" became "A promising pupil. She is keen, capable and has a careful, hard-working approach to her studies." Phrases like "capable and enthusiastic", "neat, keen and able", and "always gives of her best" cropped up regularly, and have rung true throughout my life. I'll throw myself into most things enthusiastically, roll up my sleeves and put in the effort. On the whole, I'll produce a reasonable, but unremarkable, result. It's a sound recipe for getting through life.

Another consistent thread in my teachers' assessments was reference to my happy, cheerful disposition, which ultimately earned me the "Headmistress' Prize" in my final year of primary school. Sitting in the choir stalls with my friends, fidgeting with anticipation of being set free, I daydreamed about the summer holidays as the Headmistress brought proceedings to a close with a painstakingly slow build-up to the final prize of the day. A sharp poke in the ribs from the girl next to me jolted me back as I heard the Head describe "a girl who's always smiling" and my friend whispering, "It's you!" Then, I felt the shock of hearing my name read out. I don't think I'd ever won anything before, and my little chest puffed with pride as I looked over at Mum and Dad, beaming with delight and more than a bit of surprise. It was an early lesson that positivity is rewarded. I wasn't the smartest, fastest or strongest – but I worked hard and stayed positive. I learned that day it was a gift that could take me places.

I was blessed with a positive outlook on life – a natural-born optimist. When my Mum was pregnant, my parents decided that I would be named Hannah if I were a girl.

However, when I arrived, they took one look at me and saw something that made them think I was not a Hannah but a Felicity. I can only assume it was baby wind forcing a smile-like grimace, rather than that I was a particularly advanced baby who came out laughing. Either way, Felicity – meaning "happiness" – I became, and it's a name that I've generally managed to live up to.

I've also wondered whether being labelled "happiness" shaped me – that I grew into the name and, over the years, subconsciously chose to embrace a positive outlook. Part nature, part nurture. Mum and Dad used to call me their "little ray of sunshine", and I still have a birthday card they gave me for my 7th birthday with "Little Miss Sunshine" written on the front. This attitude or instinct has held me in good stead over the years. Yes, on occasion, it can lead to disappointment when hopeless optimism is rewarded with a less favourable outcome, but on the whole, it's served me well to be an optimist. I'd rather be happy most of the time, and disappointed occasionally, than eternally anticipating the worst.

My family environment was the perfect breeding ground for a happy-go-lucky little girl, and I don't underestimate the significant influence that my parents had, and continue to have, on me. Regardless of what was happening in the world around us, Mum and Dad's enduring positivity that everything would work out, which was deeply rooted in their faith, protected us from adversity. Dad would often say, "Everything happens for a reason," and that's a mantra that has carried me through life, too. Even at the very end of his life, when he was receiving palliative care at home, he remained positive and selfless. He reflected on how lucky he'd been to share over 50 years with Mum and the joy our family life had brought them. Mum's strength, courage and ability to support others through that difficult time, despite carrying the burden of grief, remains a source of inspiration and wonder.

Kindling My Competitive Edge

As I moved through my teenage years, a cooperative approach to sport transitioned into more of an active interest, fueled by my competitive edge. Being "quite good" at most things gave me confidence and motivation to be better than "quite good." I learned that working hard, whether academically or in sports, produced results, encouraging me to work harder. During the early days of sixth form, I ditched the standard school sports to join a little group of trailblazers and try my hand at rowing.

Pip and I went to a girls' school, while James attended the partner boys' school in the same town. Rowing was one of the main sports in the boys' school. We'd regularly see the boys' school 1st V111 strut their stuff through town, looking dashing and more than a little out of reach. Taking up rowing seemed like an excellent way of getting a little bit closer to the boys, although sometimes a little too close for comfort.

I've always been on the small side of average, so I do not have a typical rower's build. For that reason, I started my rowing life as a Cox, sitting in the stern of the boat, barking instructions at the crew and attempting to steer a reasonable course. I thought I was getting the hang of it, until one day my steering let me down and we found ourselves veering off course into the path of the oncoming boys' 1st V111. I managed to execute the rowing equivalent of a hand-break turn, narrowly avoiding a collision, but wounding my pride in the process. Lesson learned: Be careful what you wish for. It was not an advisable way to get close to the boys.

Pushing aside my wounded pride, I persevered but soon became disillusioned with the prospect of coxing. Rowing, even at school, is demanding in the training stakes, requiring lots of early morning starts, come rain, shine or freezing conditions. I realised that being a Cox meant all the downsides of the early starts with none of the upsides. Sitting on your bottom, making small adjustments to the steering "strings," is not conducive to either getting fit or keeping warm through the winter months. So, I swapped my little seat in the stern for a sliding seat in the bow and got to grips with mastering the art of rowing and building my strength and fitness.

A rite of passage for novice rowers at school was learning our trade in heavy wooden sculling boats before being let loose in the sleeker, much more expensive, carbon-fibre racing boats. I did my time, but it was not without incident. I remember one outing in particular, for all of the wrong reasons. As I cautiously made my way down the beautiful River Wye in one of these not-so-fondly named "tubs," just starting to find my flow with the blades slicing through water and birdsong in the background, my trance-like state was broken by the sound of an approaching crew going full tilt, complete with their Cox's frantic shouts invading the peace.

Fearing I was about to be run down, and with panic rising in my chest, I turned to look over my shoulder, upsetting my fragile balance. The boat wobbled, and, forgetting all the rules of sculling, I threw down my oars in a panic and promptly capsized, resurfacing coughing, spluttering and looking like a drowned rat. To add insult to injury, the boys' 1st V111 had to abandon their sprint while their coach fished me out of the water into his launch and dragged my boat back to the boat house to dry off. Despite the chill of the water, my cheeks stung red with embarrassment. It was a lesson learned the hard way.

It was hardly a promising start for a future ocean rower, but what doesn't kill you makes you stronger, and lessons learned in adversity tend to stay with you for life. Decades later, mid-Atlantic, I remembered that particular lesson when, panicked by a flurry of flying fish (okay, maybe just one), I threw myself off my seat, landing, legs akimbo, in the bottom of the boat. I was wedged between my seat and the gunnels, but gripped tightly to my oars as I'd been taught to do. With the sound of panicked flapping wings now even closer to my head, and no immediate escape route, all I could do was laugh at the predicament I had thrown myself into.

Rowing at school was my first real experience of pushing myself hard physically, and I found it was something I not only enjoyed but was actually good at. For the first time, training was a serious and competitive business, but also a collaborative effort. The goal was a seat in the 1st V111, and having started late and being smaller than most, it was an uphill battle, but one I relished. Feeling like the underdog was a new experience that I embraced and used to my advantage. Nobody had great expectations of me, so achieving anything felt like a great accomplishment. Without the weight of expectation or pressure, I could train freely, slightly under the radar. I loved the feeling of my heart beating in my chest, my lungs screaming, and my legs burning, and I saw positive results – lifting heavier weights, better erg scores, nippier, and longer training runs. I also loved the discipline, structure and camaraderie of training – the early starts, the sense of achievement from working out before school, the variety of technical, strength and conditioning training, and being part of something that felt a little like a "movement."

Alongside learning the mechanics of rowing, my attitude to training translated into finding myself competitive and in with a shot at a seat in the boat. Lots of us had the technical ability to row, so crunch time was the erg test. Who had the strength and determination to get the best scores? A minute on an erg when you're going as hard as you can is torture, and it felt like I nearly killed myself that day in my effort to post a high score. We had rowing machines lined up outside the boathouse and took turns to time-trial against the machine over a set distance, encouraged and surrounded by the rest of the squad. I can't remember my time now, but it felt like a lifetime, the meters going down painfully slowly as my muscles became increasingly exhausted. My lungs felt like they'd explode, and I struggled to get enough breath to keep going. I was far from being the best, but it was enough to earn me a coveted seat in the boat. That was one of my first tastes of the pride you get when you achieve something you thought was out of reach.

Although relatively short-lived, I loved my rowing days at school. I loved getting fit and strong, pushing myself physically, being part of a team, and the collective competitive spirit we shared – sometimes competing against each other for a place in the boat, but usually together. Much like the rest of my school days, we achieved a moderate degree of success, winning some races, losing others, going on to represent Wales and becoming Junior National Champions.

I look back on school rowing as formative. It was the foundation of my passion for physical challenge and exercise, which became integral to my identity, and a life lesson in the rewards of working hard. But much as I loved rowing, that is where I left it for 25 years.

The Seeds of Adventure Were Planted

I took a year "out" after leaving school, breaking the rowing habit. Although I missed it, by the time I started University in Nottingham, I'd convinced myself that rowing and enjoying uni were entirely incompatible, so I opted to throw myself into the social side of student life instead. Sport took a back seat during my uni days; I dabbled in aerobics (it was the 90s) and a spot of running, but my time was mainly spent having fun and doing enough to earn myself a solid 2:1.

After uni, I followed the crowd and moved to London to start my graduate role in one of the "big banks." The move to London and earning what I thought was a decent wage was the catalyst for returning to proper exercise. I joined a local gym and became a regular, rekindling my love of training and pushing myself. But it soon started to feel a bit pointless without a goal. I needed to find something to work towards.

I had continued to do a bit of running when I moved to London, and during a holiday in Greece, after taking a few wrong turns, I managed to clock up a couple of 90-minute runs. Realising I could run a reasonable distance, and inspired by a marathon-running uni friend, Adriano, I decided to go big and enter the London Marathon. It was a terrifying prospect. I now know so many people who have run marathons, but when I entered, I only knew a couple of people mad enough to run 26 miles, so it felt like a massive stretch. The fear of the unknown even penetrated my sleep. On more than one occasion, I woke, heart racing, damp with the cold sweat of fear after dreaming about the impending doom. Could I do it?

But that fear became my motivation to train hard. I knew that if I was going to finish the race, I had to put in the work, and I was determined to finish the race. But I also knew that if I put in the effort, I could finish the race and do it in a time I could be proud of. Through rowing, I learned that effort is rewarded and that I had the self-discipline and motivation to push myself.

I found a training plan, decked myself out in new running kit so that I felt like a proper runner, and got down to the business of marathon training. My fear of the challenge ahead meant I didn't miss a single training run. I followed the plan religiously, usually going a little bit further or longer than it said for good measure. And I made progress. I loved clocking up the miles, getting stronger and faster, and ticking off the training runs. Following a plan was an easy way for me to break down this huge, frightening goal into daily, achievable steps, and it gave me the structure and discipline I'd missed from my rowing days.

I told my friends and family that I wanted to finish in under 4 hours and 30 minutes – a very respectable time for a first-time marathon runner. But I set myself a sub-4-hour target. I'd trained for it, so I knew I could do it. All sorts of people offered me advice to start slowly and not be too ambitious, and I nodded politely and ignored it. I had my race plan, and I stuck to it. I knew that persistence, determination and hard work would pay off. I ran a negative split (the second half marginally faster than the first half). I managed to run through the "wall" that most runners find difficult to push through. And, as I turned the corner into the final straight, a man running alongside said, "Come on, we're going to be under 4 hours!" It was all I needed to pump my lead-like legs a little harder for the final few hundred meters, emotions rising as the crowds clapped and cheered and the famous finish line grew closer. I crossed the line in 3 hours, 52 minutes. As a marshall handed me my medal and foil blanket, I was surprised to feel a few tears stinging my eyes and a lump forming in my throat. I was delighted, relieved, exhausted and just a teeny, weeny bit smug. When others had said, "You can't," I'd said, "I can." And I did.

Looking back, I can see the pattern of tools I've consistently used to build my mental resilience. During both the hard yards of training and the latter stages of the marathon itself, when your legs are tired and you start to question whether you can keep going, I'd rationalise and reframe the task still ahead. It wasn't the 21st, 22nd, 23rd mile and so on. In my head, it was just the equivalent of a short training run, and that's something I knew I could do. I'd also think about all the training I had put in, which gave me the confidence that I could do it.

The marathon was my first foray into endurance events, and from there, I didn't look back. Knowing I could do things that most people wouldn't even contemplate made me want to do them more. It gave me a massive sense of achievement and pride, filling me with self-belief and curiosity. If I can run a marathon, then what else can I do?

After the marathon came cycling, which transitioned into triathlons. I replaced public transport with commuting on two wheels or on foot, often running the 12 miles from my Wimbledon home to the office in Canary Wharf. Colleagues thought I was mad, but commuting became an important part of my training.

The stumbling block to start with was swimming. I was a reasonably competent swimmer and could swim endless lengths of a pool doing breaststroke, but I needed to crack front crawl to compete in triathlons. I saw it as an opportunity to gain a new skill, so I booked a few private lessons in the local swimming pool and relearned how to swim front crawl. Once again, the fear of being unable to finish a triathlon spurred me on. I found a triathlon swimming training plan, and I got stuck in. It was torture to start with, and I'd be gasping for breath at the end of each length, heart pounding against my chest, wondering how on earth I was going to manage 1.5km. Slowly but surely, my stroke, breathing and stamina improved, and soon enough I was happily gliding up and down the pool or lido, feeling like a proper swimmer.

My 30s were characterised by training and competing in triathlons, spurred on by my friends Emma, Lucy and Lou. We'd spend weekends cycling to Windsor or the Surrey Hills, with obligatory stops for coffee and cake, and hours ploughing up and down Tooting Bec Lido with other early-morning, wetsuit-clad swimmers. We even ventured into longer-distance events, including an Ironman 70.3 and the Great Kindrochit Quadrathlon – a brilliant, crazy, 12-hour effort in and around Loch Tay, ending with slicing open a watermelon with a sword. I can highly recommend it if you're after an endurance event with a difference. It may sound serious, but the emphasis was on sociability and the experience (for me, anyway). While I usually did reasonably well, it was not about being the strongest or the fastest.

I was motivated by challenging myself to do things that most people wouldn't attempt, which scared me and pushed me to work hard. I loved the process of working towards a goal. I relished the journey and everything it taught me: from overcoming challenges and building new skills to the steady progress of daily effort and the joy of surpassing my goals.

Beyond anything, these years and events taught me that with the right mindset and hard work, ordinary, unremarkable, smaller-than-average people like me can achieve extraordinary things.

Chapter 2
The Dodgy Hip

Somehow, between working and training for various multi-disciplinary endurance events, I managed to find time for a little bit of dating.

A little bit of dating turned into a lot of dating. After three years of consistently demonstrating my eligibility as a life partner, in April 2012, on the day we completed the purchase of our house, Paul proposed. He'd hoped this might buy him time before actually having to organise a wedding, but life had other ideas.

We were in our mid-thirties, so we were hardly in the first flush of youth, and my body clock was ticking like a time bomb. Some might call it impeccable planning, some might call it carelessness. I like to think of it as a very happy accident, but a few days after saying "yes," I discovered I was pregnant. I think my body had sensed that everything was falling into place nicely to accommodate a child, and decided we needed to get a wriggle on. Although we hadn't planned for it to happen quite then, we got over the momentary shock and looked forward to the impending arrival of our baby.

Unfortunately for Paul, it also precipitated the conversation around when we'd get married. Our options were to do it quickly or wait until sometime after the birth, but I didn't fancy our chances of finding the energy to organise a wedding with a young baby in tow, so we decided on the shotgun approach.

Wasting no time, we got to work. A few busy weeks later, during an unseasonally wet July in 2012, we were married, my slightly thickening waist more or less concealed by my corseted dress. It was a wonderful, joyous, if sober (for me) day, complete with a sniggering congregation as the vicar professed his hope that our marriage would be blessed with children. I spent the following few months trying to avoid seeing the vicar, even hiding in the potato snack aisle of the local Coop, to avoid him noticing the increasingly visible bump and putting two and two together.

The Transition to Parenthood

We were incredibly fortunate to sail through the majority of my pregnancy. I loved being pregnant, seeing my body change to accommodate a new life, feeling the little "bubble" movements gradually change into palpable kicks and marvelling at my tummy growing and stretching like an inflating balloon. Physically, I felt brilliant. I genuinely felt like I was blooming and flourishing with the new life within me. I also felt immeasurably blessed and thankful to be given this gift of motherhood. As a woman in my mid-thirties, I knew that my fertility was probably entering a steep decline, and having seen close friends struggle to conceive, and others suffer horribly through pregnancy, becoming a mother and enjoying pregnancy was not something I took for granted. I counted myself lucky every day for the privilege, and concluded it was well worth the label of "geriatric" assigned to me (and all women over a certain age) by the NHS.

While wedding planning and impending parenthood had ended my triathlon exploits, it wasn't an excuse to abandon exercise altogether, and I modified my regimen to accommodate the bump. I switched spin and weights for swimming, running and static cycling, and kept it up throughout. I was on my turbo trainer in the garage when my midwife called to tell me she wanted me to be induced a few days early due to suspected pre-eclampsia.

Fortunately, it was only a minor hiccup and a precautionary intervention into an otherwise textbook pregnancy. (If you ignore the geriatric element.) The hospital birth was not the romantic, wonderful experience I had naively imagined or hoped for. Paul described the aftermath as being like a scene from *Reservoir Dogs*. Nonetheless, little Samuel Robert Ashley arrived safely, and mercifully for me anyway, a bijou

7 lb 3 oz. He'd also arrived in time for Dad to be able to proudly announce the news at Church, before bombing up the motorway with Mum to pay their respects. Being the last of their children to become parents, I think Sam's birth brought Mum and Dad immense pride, joy and a sense of relief and completeness.

We took to parenthood like ducks to water. With the benefit of hindsight, Sam was an easy baby after a difficult birth. He rarely cried and gorged himself on breast milk for hours on end, affording me ample opportunity to binge Netflix. He very soon became a ludicrously fat, happy little boy. Within a couple of weeks, he'd rocketed up the weight chart to the 98th percentile while I checked and double-checked with the midwife that you can't overfeed a breast-fed baby. Dad declared me to be the human equivalent of a Jersey milking cow.

Sam was so tired from feeding that he also became a good sleeper, at least during the day, and I used the time while he slept to get myself fit again. When he was around 5 weeks old, I ventured out for my first run, which felt amazing and liberating. But after stretching off, I noticed some pain in my right hip. I didn't think much of it, assuming I'd probably strained a ligament from exercising and stretching too much, too soon after giving birth. I've never been a stickler for following doctors' orders.

Finding My Superpower

My hip pain continued. It was irritating rather than debilitating, a niggle that would catch every so often. It didn't stop me from doing anything, so I carried on. But after a couple of months of the pain not receding, I decided to see a physiotherapist. I was given a programme of exercises, which I diligently followed, and kept returning to the physio, who was flummoxed by my lack of progress.

The pain became increasingly frequent and more inconvenient over time. It was the kind of pain that would literally stop me in my tracks, and when you're trying to prevent small children from running amok around car parks or crossing the road, it's far from ideal. The range of movement in my hip also became increasingly limited. Getting on and off a bike was tricky. I didn't have the lateral movement to swing my leg over the crossbar, and would have to lay the bike on the ground before standing over the frame and raising it. Equally challenging was sitting cross-legged. Ordinarily, as an adult, I could live without that, but if you've ever frequented baby groups, you'll appreciate that chairs are a luxury and know that sitting cross-legged on the floor is tantamount to law. Ben, baby number two, came along during this period, so baby groups stayed part of daily life.

Eventually, after around three years of intermittently returning to the physio, with a slow but steady deterioration in my condition, I finally accepted that the inconvenience of the pain was now greater than the inconvenience of seeking further intervention. The physio and I decided to call it a day and get a referral to the big guns – the surgeons.

After the requisite scans, I was summoned back to the hospital to await sentencing by an orthopaedic surgeon. Sitting opposite the surgeon, I watched with curiosity as he pointed at the indecipherable images on his screen, waiting for him to send me packing back to the physio for yet more glute strengthening exercises. It was with some surprise that I heard him unleash his verdict: "Your hip is 100% screwed."

I sat bolt upright in the chair, sensing this was not a job for the physio. An initial frown gave way to a wry smile; his words validated the pain I'd been experiencing. I hadn't been exaggerating the issue, and I hadn't been slacking on the physio front. He pointed out an extra hook of bone that was growing, grinding into the joint and accounting for the acute stabbing pain. Then there was the almost total eradication of cartilage and the inflammation of arthritis. He told me that 99% of people with a hip in that condition couldn't even walk down the road, so he was amazed that I could still run for an hour or so. It's not that it didn't hurt, but I chose to push through the pain because the gains were greater. No pain, no gain. Right?

So at the ripe old age of 39, I was told I needed a full, right hip replacement. Ball, socket – the lot.

I stared at him, mouth gaping like a goldfish, lost for words, as his words sank in. Hip replacements were for older people. If not quite in the first flush of youth, I was certainly not ready to be consigned to the scrap heap. I felt like my head was stuffed with cotton wool, as a jumble of thoughts jostled for attention. What? How? When? Could I still exercise with a new hip? Could I run around with the children?

Contemplating this unlikely turn of events, and wondering how this was all going to work with a baby and toddler on my hands, he told me to carry on until the pain started to impact my life unreasonably.

It was hardly the diagnosis I expected or wanted as a young mother of two small children. And yet, as I drove away from the hospital that day, and the initial shock of the diagnosis wore off, I was bemused to find myself smiling, and almost giddy with a feeling that I can really only describe as elation. Odd, I know. It was so odd that I mulled it over and realised it was for two reasons.

Firstly, when he told me that most people in my condition couldn't even walk, yet I could still run, I translated this in my head as "I'm nails." I thought, "I'm tougher than most and can take more pain than most." And that made me feel good. It felt like my superpower. It was as if he'd given me a label, confirming all of my experiences through my marathon and triathlon days.

And secondly, I'd realised there was a solution to my pain. After all the years of trekking to see the physio, with hours of fruitless strength and mobility exercises but a continual deterioration in my condition, I finally had an answer. My hip was irredeemably wrecked; no amount of physio or exercising could make it better, but my lovely surgeon, with his sledgehammer and drill, could. It was a case of going out with the old and in with the new.

One of my first questions for the surgeon was what I could do with a new hip, and his answer became instrumental in the future of my story. He said, "You might not want to run a marathon, but you can do pretty much anything else."

So a new hip would give me a new lease of life, opening doors that I'd thought were shut, allowing me to pursue more wacky events, if I wished. It was a way for me to get back to doing the things I loved again and regain a part of my identity that I thought I'd lost. It was a way for me to be me again. Yes, there may be the temporary challenges of surgery and months of rehabilitation to follow, but a hip replacement represented an opportunity that was so much more powerful for me than the inconvenience of the surgery.

When I reflect on different times in my life when I've faced challenges, I realise that the uncertainty or the unknown is the hardest to cope with. But once I have the answers, know what challenge I'm dealing with and can look it square in the face, I have the foundations to make a plan. You can't fight an enemy you can't see. But finally, I could see this one. I'd seen what I was dealing with in black and white on my surgeon's computer screen. Together, my surgeon and I could formulate a plan of attack.

The surgeon's suggestion, to go away and come back when it was unreasonably impacting my life, was rather vague. What did "unreasonable impact" mean?

So I limped on, literally and metaphorically, for another 3 years, when our third and final child, Grace, came along. My hip condition continued to worsen over this period. It would spontaneously give way with increasing regularity, and my range of lateral movement became pathetic. Even swinging my leg into the car was painful. When Grace turned one, and the fog of baby days was beginning to lift, I decided enough was enough, and once again knocked on my surgeon's door.

"I'm back, I think it's now unreasonably impacting my life," I told him. He replied that he'd expected me back after a few months, not three years. Well, I am nails, I thought. Plus, I'd wanted a third child, and I wouldn't let a dodgy hip get in the way of that.

Fortunately, hip technology had advanced within the intervening period, becoming much more personalised. The surgeon told me with great delight about the 3-D-printed ceramic hip he'd make for me, exactly replicating my old one, presumably without the extra hooks of bone that were growing.

"When do you want to come in?" he asked. " Could I fit you in in three weeks?" Fortunately, thanks to private health insurance, I could pick the date of my surgery, which meant I could work it around our busy family life.

Three weeks was far too soon – I didn't want to be on crutches through the summer – so we settled on a date a few months away in early September, once Ben, our second, had started school and Grace would be more mobile at nearly two. The challenge with a new hip is bending past 90 degrees and lifting heavy weights, and Grace had followed the family trend of being distinctly larger and chubbier than the average baby. So, bending and lifting heavy weights was something I did a lot. If I could wait until she was nearly two and mobile, the worst of the lifting would hopefully be over. I didn't want to run the risk of dislocating my lovely new hip.

Turning Adversity Into Opportunity

September came, we settled Ben into school, and I into a lovely room in the local private hospital for three nights of rest and recuperation. And honestly, that's how I saw it. As a parent of three young children, life is hard work. It's a constant juggling act, with barely a minute's peace and slim chance of an uninterrupted night's sleep. So, three nights in a private hospital – with posh coffee and shortbread at the press of a button, someone else cooking and delivering my meals, and an extensive Netflix watch list – felt like a holiday.

My surgery went well; the 100% screwed hip was hacked out and the shiny new ceramic one shoe-horned in. As I emerged from deep sedation in the recovery room, the surgeon reassured me that all had gone well and that my hip was one of the worst he'd ever seen. Once again, a little puff of pride welled in my chest, and I mentally polished my "nails" badge. It's funny how we use our perspective to interpret things differently.

My mini-break in hospital wasn't quite the holiday I'd imagined, but it was pretty good. I was horribly sick from the heady mix of drugs, but once the offending opiates were out of my system, it was onwards and upwards. I was up on my feet and shuffling around the following morning, the first tentative weight-bearing step leading to the next, and so on. I learned how to climb stairs and became a frequent flyer around the hospital corridors. The physio was delighted by my speedy progress, remarking that most patients lack enough strength in their upper body to push themselves up to sitting so they can get their legs out of bed. Having this kind of surgery as a relatively young person was not something to lament or a reason to feel sorry for myself. It was a huge advantage, and one I was immensely grateful for.

Rehab continued to go well when I went back home, and soon I walked around for longer each day without crutches, building the strength around my new joint. I was desperate to get back to exercise again, so I diligently did my physio exercises, doing a little more, rather than less, every day. The physio was delighted with my progress, allowing me back on a cross trainer for light exercise after just three weeks.

From there, there was no looking back. While I remained cautious about the risk of dislocation and avoided high-risk movements, I got back into a reasonably normal training routine. I loved exercising without pain or fear of pain again. It was early days, but the relief of being pain-free was significant, and I was already reaping the rewards of the "challenge" of surgery. I was starting to feel like me again.

The most frustrating part of this episode was being unable to drive for over a month. With three small children on our hands, and living on the outskirts of a small village, driving is a lifeline and a many-times daily activity. I hate being dependent on others and feeling like I'm not pulling my weight, but I had to accept help with the driving and ferrying. Paul, my parents, neighbours and friends rallied around, and Paul and I were grateful to have this support network around us.

The children fared brilliantly during my short spell in hospital, buoyed by the excitement of a new school/pre-school term and having Granny and Poppa on hand to answer every beck and call. Arriving home after my surgery, they were intrigued by my slower progress around the house and Sam, in particular, was delighted with the addition of the crutches to his toy stash. He alternated between stubbornly insisting he could use them for their designated purpose and zooming around on one as a broomstick. Inevitably, this meant they were often nowhere near when I needed to use them. Necessity is the mother of invention, and I quickly learned to get around without them.

Grace, who was almost two, was too young to understand what was going on. It tugged at my heartstrings and took all my resolve not to respond to her outstretched arms, imploring expression and hopeful "up, up" requests. Paul became adept at anticipating the stand-off, and would swoop in to the rescue. Fortunately, Grace adored Paul and was generally happy to be hoisted up to his giddier heights.

As much as surgery and rehab had been inconvenient and painful, I knew it was something I needed to do to regain my mobility and reclaim some of the old me again. I'm a big believer in silver linings. I could see that the silver lining in this particular case was being able to live life without stabbing pain again, which meant I'd be able to exercise properly, play with my kids without fearing collapse and save them from running into the road.

Mindset is everything when it comes to tackling challenges, and seeing surgery as something positive rather than negative, as a necessary stepping stone to pain-free days, allowed me to approach it in the right way. There was a bright, silver lining to this particular cloud, opening up a world of opportunities.

Little did I know where these opportunities would take me.

Chapter 3
Feel the Fear and Do It Anyway

During my rehabilitation from hip surgery, our family's attention turned to an extreme adventure that Pip's husband, David, was about to embark on. He was part of a five-person crew taking part in the Talisker Whisky Atlantic Challenge, a.k.a. "The World's Toughest Row." It was an epic 3,000-mile unsupported rowing race from La Gomera in the Canary Islands to Antigua in the Caribbean.

I'd first heard about this race a year or so before, when they entered the race and concluded he was absolutely bonkers. The idea of voluntarily putting yourself in a tiny boat, in the middle of a massive, unpredictable ocean, for an indeterminate period, was terrifying to me, sending shudders down my spine. I had visions of "The Perfect Storm" in my head – rather you than me, I thought.

Rowing the Atlantic had been a lifelong dream for David. Aged seven, he'd read a book about the first ever successful

Atlantic crossing in a rowing boat, and had decided then that it was something he wanted to do. To his immense credit, he made it happen.

David and his crew, The Felix Five, got on with the job of training while the rest of us went about our lives. I didn't think much more about it until the time came for him to say goodbye to Pip and their four children, and head off to the race start in La Gomera.

It was early December 2019. We were getting ready for a family Christmas with my parents, which would be a little different this year without David. Naturally, over the Christmas period, there was a lot of chat about the row, and Dad embraced the sport of "dot watching" – tracking the dot that represented the Felix Five – every four hours, day and night, as it made its way slowly across 3,000 miles of Atlantic. We even had a couple of calls from David while we were all together, and the live updates from the ocean added to the excitement.

Dad's enthusiasm was infectious, and when we returned to our Oxfordshire home after the Christmas break, I continued to track David and the crew, becoming increasingly hooked by the stream of race updates posted on social media. But it was watching him finish the race live on Facebook, which was the defining, pivotal moment for me.

He was due to finish in the middle of the night, UK time, so I set my alarm, put my headphones in and tuned into Facebook Live to see them finish. As I sat there in bed, watching this little boat emerge from the darkness to cross the finish line and seeing the look of sheer elation on the wild-looking faces of the crew, my heart began to race. A tingle of excitement spread up my spine and rippled through my hair. After 41 days at sea, over Christmas and New Year, they had achieved something extraordinary: a feat accomplished by fewer people than have travelled to space. I blinked back tears as I watched them achieve a life-long dream, and remember thinking to myself, "If I feel like this, thousands of miles away, sitting in bed, what must it be like to be in that boat, crossing the line and knowing you are one of very few people to have experienced that?"

I couldn't imagine what it must feel like, but I recalled the sense of achievement and pride I'd felt when I'd completed challenges, albeit on a much more modest scale – the Ironman 70.3, quadrathlon and London marathon. I concluded it must be something very special, blowing everything else out of the water. The seed was planted at that moment, and I knew I wanted to experience it for myself…one day.

Opportunity Calls

Over the following days, the thought kept coming back into my head, and I'd push it away. But I started thinking about how I could make it happen and when. I rationalised that 5 to 10 years was probably a "reasonable" timeframe, when the children would be older and more independent, but I would still be young enough to do it. It felt like I was taking a sensible approach to a nonsensical adventure.

But life rarely goes entirely according to plan. Just a few days later, the phone rang, and it was Pip, back from her trip to Antigua to see David finish. After the usual "How was it?" pleasantries, she cut to the chase. "Anyway, Dids, I've got a boat. Do you want to row the Atlantic with me?" Standing in our sitting room doorway, my hand trembled as I gripped the phone, and butterflies in my stomach radiated a warm glow that coloured my cheeks. An involuntary smile broke my lips before I responded with jumbled questions. "How have you got a boat?" "When?" "Are you being serious?" These questions were buying me time to think.

Pip explained that she was deadly serious. The owner of Mrs Nelson, a 28-foot ocean rowing boat for David's crew, had offered to keep the boat if she wanted to form a crew. And she did.

"So, what do you think?" The words that came out of my mouth did not reflect what my physical reaction was telling me, but it seemed like the "correct" response to such a ridiculous proposal. I told Pip I couldn't possibly do it, citing some objectively valid reasons why not: "I've just had a hip replacement and the kids are too young. I can't leave them for that long!" The race would mean two months away from home. Most would concede that these were fairly robust reasons for saying "no."

However, Pip can be pretty persuasive, and she's not the type to take no for an answer. She swiftly dismissed my feeble excuses, saying:

"Stop giving me reasons why you can't, and start giving me reasons why you can."

As she's an executive coach, I'm pretty sure it's not the first time she's pulled that one out of the bag. But it resonated and is a lesson that will stay with me for life. Those words lit a spark in me. When I put the phone down, I was grinning from ear to ear with fire in my belly, because I knew I would say *yes*.

Turning My Can'ts Into Cans

Could I do it? I don't think I questioned my ability to do it for one second, and I don't know where that self-belief comes from. Perhaps my experience during my school days of working hard and seeing the progress and rewards had taught me that I could do anything I worked for. But I'd also seen others do it before me. At that point, around 200 women in the world had rowed an ocean. So if they could do it, then why not me? And seeing it done by David, someone like me, made it not just possible, but probable.

It wasn't just a question of whether I had the physical and mental capacity to do it. I had my family to consider. The impact on Paul and the children would be huge, and it was as much about our collective ability to do it as it was about my desire and ability to do it.

Still gripping the phone, absent-mindedly turning it over and over in my hand, I performed slow laps around the sitting room, distracted by the thoughts flying through my mind. Was it crazy to even consider doing it? Was it reckless? Would Paul think I was an irresponsible parent if I broached the subject? How would the children cope without me? Would the emotional burden be too much for them? What would other people think? My sensible, rational brain tried to bury the idea, but my heart was already on the journey.

I had to at least have the conversation with Paul and make the decision together. I hate confrontation or conflict, and more than that, I hated the idea that he might think less of me, so I was nervous about how the conversation would go. Taking a deep breath and throwing caution to the wind, I sidestepped my usual procrastination and jumped straight in.

"Pip's asked me if I want to row the Atlantic with her," I gabbled, relieved to have aired the words.

Paul looked up and asked, "Do you want to?" I think he already knew the answer.

"Yes," I replied. "But it would mean being away for two months, and I know that's a huge ask of you and the kids."

To Paul's huge credit (and my immense relief) he said in an admittedly resigned tone: "Well, this can either be a long conversation or a short one, so let's make it a short one."

I had been expecting some push-back: maybe a reasoned debate or impassioned plea to rethink the wisdom of this endeavour. We had three young dependents, after all. It wasn't just about me or what I wanted to do. It wasn't like I was suggesting I'd go on a girls' weekend. I was asking if he'd take sole responsibility at home, so that I could disappear for a couple of months to embark on an extraordinary and outwardly risky adventure. This would mean a very significant impact on our little family. I would be away for Christmas and New Year, a busy, chaotic time for families; the children would still be young (four, six and eight), needing a lot of hands-on care, and they'd also be dealing with the emotional fallout of their Mummy being away for a long time. And I was also asking him if he'd be okay with one of the people he loves most in the world and the mother of his children, attempting something which comes with the real, albeit improbable, risk of not returning. I knew I was asking for a lot.

So, I have tremendous respect, admiration and gratitude for how Paul approached not only my request but also his role throughout the challenge – from supporting me through training for nearly two years to the two months of solo-parenting while I was away.

I know there are lots of solo parents out there doing it all on their own for all sorts of reasons, without any recognition. But we are a team, and we had a choice.

There's no way I could have contemplated the challenge without Paul's support. I needed him, the children needed him, and he gave us 110%. That's not to say he was doing backflips with joy at the prospect, but he was selflessly all-in, fully committed to his significant part in this extraordinary adventure.

With Paul's support and reassurance that he and the children would cope, it didn't take me long to find my "cans." I knew that the only thing standing in my way now was me, and the power to say yes lay firmly in my hands. "I can't leave the kids for that long," was all about me and the guilt I would bear for going away over Christmas. They would adjust quickly to me being away, Father Christmas would still visit, and soon enough, they'd be looking forward to a holiday in Antigua.

My shiny new ceramic hip wasn't an excuse to say no, either. It was a reason to say yes, a reason why I *could* do it. I was pain-free, with a fully functioning hip that had opened up a world of opportunity.

I Can, and I Will

I had my "cans," and now it was down to me to decide whether I had what it took, including the desire and motivation to do it. The ball was in my court. It's all very well thinking about doing something, having it as a little secret in my head to fuel daydreams. But when the opportunity landed in my lap, I had a decision to make. Could I, should I, would I say yes and commit?

I'm not always great at making decisions – I can dither and pontificate, agonising over the options. But this one came easily. Burning deep inside me was a flame I couldn't put out, nor did I want to. The thrill of an adventure was on the horizon, spurring me on.

This row was one of the ultimate tests of physical and mental endurance, but I knew I was capable of both. I'd demonstrated to myself through my triathlon days that I could push myself and enjoy it, and I believed I was nails. The surgeon had told me (in my head, at least)! However, an event like that cannot be achieved by ability alone. Mental resilience plays a huge role, and part of that mental resilience, I believe, is about having the motivation to do something.

I knew I was blessed with the kind of positive, "can-do" growth mindset you need to tackle challenges like this. I'd seen evidence of it on so many occasions in my life, from marathon training to my hip replacement. I always found the positives and silver linings in any situation, and I was motivated to do it.

Your ability to tackle challenges is contingent on motivation. I truly believe that we all have the ability to take on extraordinary challenges, but the difference between those who do and those who don't is motivation.

Motivation can be complex and multi-faceted.

Firstly, I was motivated to do it for myself. Having completed many "mini" endurance events in the past, I knew I was tough, but that also made me curious. I wanted to know how far I could push myself. Would I reach my limits, mentally and physically? How would I cope with the fear of the ocean when things got really tough? Could I conquer my fear? How would I react when face to face with the waves, my demons? Was I really as nails as I believed?

It was also an opportunity for me to reignite part of my identity. Physical challenges and adventure had defined me before having children. The reality of becoming a parent, in itself an endurance event on a totally different level, combined with a deteriorating hip, had inevitably put the kibosh on my sporting challenges. We were starting to see the light at the end of the tunnel with sleepless nights and baby days, and my new hip had given me a new lease of life, opening the door to physical challenges.

Most importantly, I was motivated to set an example for my children. I'd seen my nephews' and nieces' reactions to David rowing the Atlantic – the excitement and pride on their faces when they talked about what he was doing, how they spoke about doing it themselves as a crew of siblings one day. It was infectious and wonderful to see children not questioning their ability or right to tackle extraordinary things. I wanted to inspire my children too, to inspire them to dream big and show them that, with the right mindset and a lot of hard work, ordinary people like their Mummy can achieve extraordinary things. I wanted them to grow up free of the shackles of limiting beliefs that stop so many people from even contemplating challenges. Being a mum of boys and a girl, it was imperative to me that they grow up knowing that adventures are for boys and girls, men and women, mummies and daddies. And I could help show them that.

And then there was, I have to admit, an element of "fear of missing out." I had been conditioned, from birth, to jostle and compete with my siblings. There was no way I wanted to sit on the sidelines and watch while my *younger* sister embarked on an incredible adventure. Turning down the opportunity of a lifetime just to watch someone else do it would have gnawed away at me like an insidious disease.

But greater than the desire not to miss out was the desire not to miss out on the opportunity to do it with Pip, as a team. We'd fought like cats and dogs growing up, as many siblings do, but we'd grown incredibly close over time. Since the arrival of our seven children, there were limited opportunities to spend quality time together and have conversations that ran deeper than the practicalities of what to dish up for tea, or the logistics of transporting the crowd from A to B. The prospect of sharing this adventure, experiencing highs and lows together and getting to know each other on a completely different level was incredibly motivating.

Should I do it? That was probably the hardest question. Just because I was motivated to do it, and could do it, didn't mean I *should* do it. Although safety is paramount in the race, rowing an ocean carries an element of inherent risk, and it wasn't just me I had to think about. Paul, Sam, Ben and Grace were huge considerations. It wasn't just that it was risky, but there was also the question of how they'd cope emotionally with me being away. I was fairly sure Paul would be fine, but I'd seen how Pip's children had reacted to David rowing the Atlantic. Of course, they missed him, but it was outweighed by immense pride and excitement.

I knew it wouldn't be easy for them to be without their mum for such a long time, but I also knew that Paul would do everything he could to fill the time with love, laughter and entertainment while I was away. I hoped that any temporary heartache would be more than compensated for by what they would gain: a spirit of adventure, curiosity about the world and unlimiting self-belief.

So the crunch question. Would I do it?

A resounding, committed, *yes*. I'd turned my perfectly valid "can'ts" into "cans," and I had the curiosity, desire and motivation to do it. The flame of anticipation was already burning brightly within.

I believe that things happen for a reason, and opportunities are gifts to be taken. I had been given an incredible opportunity to do something extraordinary, and I wouldn't let it pass.

Within 24 hours of the phone ringing and Pip dangling the opportunity in front of me, I called her back and said, "Yes."

In that one small word was a huge commitment, and with it, the first and arguably most difficult step on a two-year journey to row 3,000 miles across the Atlantic to become one of fewer than 250 women to row an ocean.

I had turned the page on a new and defining chapter in my life.

Big decisions take courage. We often fear what lies ahead. But we have to learn to embrace that fear and use it as fuel.

We fear the unknown: not having all of the answers or the path clearly paved ahead. Sometimes, we just have to take a leap of faith and trust that we will find the answers and the path will become clear. Sometimes, we might not make the right decisions or we take a wrong turn. But that's okay too, because when we do that, we learn and grow.

The little, but loud, nagging voices in our head tell us we can't do something, brainwashing us with limiting beliefs. We need to silence those voices and reframe those thoughts, finding our reasons to say yes rather than excuses to say no. Perhaps we fear judgement from other people: What will people think of me wanting to leave my children over Christmas to row an ocean? At the end of the day, what matters more is how we judge ourselves, because that's something we live with every minute of every day.

Chapter 4
You Don't Have to Be Great to Start, but You Do Have to Start to Be Great

Saying "yes" to Pip set in motion nearly two years of training and preparation for our adventure. Enthusiastically encouraged by David, who felt he was living his best life again through us, we devoured every book available, watched every YouTube video and listened to every podcast to learn about this strange, niche world of ocean rowing. As we took the first tentative steps to becoming bona fide transatlantic rowers, one message came through loud and clear: The hardest part of this challenge would be getting to the start line. We shrugged it off. We had a boat, we were rowers, we'd be fine.

Then a major curveball flew in from left field. China, actually. We'd heard reports of this mysterious, highly contagious virus causing chaos in the Wuhan region of China, but it didn't register as a direct concern. China was a long way away – what did it have to do with us?

But suddenly, within a few days of agreeing to row the Atlantic, this thing called COVID-19 had become a more real threat. Boris Johnson, UK Prime Minister at the time, declared lockdown number one. Even so, we naively thought it would pass quickly and life would return to normal. How wrong we were. COVID was a curse that would punctuate our campaign almost from the day we started to the day we finally crossed the finish line in Antigua. It was a challenge that ran in parallel with our campaign from start to finish – but a challenge that, like most, came with opportunities too.

While the world around us was focused on infection rates, R rate, hospital admissions and the death toll, daily life had become limited to confinement at home with only the people in our household. But we had something else to focus on, something to distract us from the horror of what was unfolding around us. Our Atlantic campaign was like a beacon of hope, a light at the end of the tunnel, which provided a purpose, a focus, a reason to get up every day and train, a reason to keep moving forward even within the limitations of this strange new world we had been thrown into. It was a reason to be positive, to feel excitement and anticipation, to feel hope for the future rather than despair for the present. And when, like millions of other parents, we were frazzled and frustrated, tearing our hair out and run ragged by the impossible task of trying to juggle working from home with home schooling three young children (while fighting a losing battle with cabin fever), the prospect of being out on the Atlantic, thousands of miles removed from all of that, was glorious.

COVID also bought us time, that precious commodity we invariably want more of. With offices closed and working from home becoming the "new normal," the time we once spent commuting was now time we could spend training. I wanted to minimise the impact of training on family life wherever possible. I knew there would be a huge impact on them while I was away for the race itself, but I didn't want their lives to be dominated by the row for the two years leading up to that point. So, whenever I could, I did my physical training early in the morning before the children woke up. It was a time, thanks to COVID, that was no longer taken up by getting ready for the morning commute to work.

So, working within the confines and leveraging the opportunities of COVID, we set to work making this hare-brained plan something closer to a reality. The first task was to put together a crew of four and find two other women brave or bonkers enough to do it with us. It was easier than we thought (maybe we all had the same need to escape from lockdown), and we had five or six keen to join the fray. But as the initial novelty and thrill of the adventure turned to the reality of making it happen – and the reality of what it would mean to be away from our children for nearly two months – there was, inevitably, some flux within the crew. By the time autumn came, and with it our first outing in our boat, Mrs Nelson, we had our four intrepid, excited, aspiring transatlantic rowers.

We had our crew, and next, we needed a crew name. Aside from being brave and a little bonkers, we were all mothers who wanted to inspire our children. So we focused on this as our central theme. During some textbook brainstorming via WhatsApp, I had a rare lightbulb moment, and The Mothership was coined.

While COVID, with its lockdowns, bubbles, social distancing and tiers, thwarted our ability to get out in the boat and start learning how to row an ocean practically, we threw ourselves into the many other workstreams involved in rowing an ocean. It proved to be quite a feat of project management. From sponsorship, branding and PR to objective setting, training courses, team dynamics, and of course, physical training, we had our work cut out.

There's a lot more to rowing an ocean than actually rowing an ocean. But life and experience are wonderful teachers. While being "mature" compared to most crews, with age comes experience, connections and a certain degree of know-how – and these were most definitely our advantage. We all had professional backgrounds and networks of contacts, which proved incredibly helpful when it came to the business side of rowing an ocean. As working parents, we had juggling down to a fine art and so were not fazed by adding a few more jobs into the mix and fitting more into a day than seemed humanly possible.

One thing that particularly struck me throughout our ocean rowing adventure was the kindness of people – strangers, professional networks, friends and family. I was pleasantly surprised by the willingness of so many people to rally around and support us when they had no skin in the game. Perhaps heightened by the way COVID had limited our horizons, our ocean row seemed to spark a light in so many people and a desire to be part of the journey with us. It took us by surprise; it was heartwarming and wonderful. The Mothership was about far more than the four of us in the boat. We had a small army of supporters who each played an important role in our adventure, from boat maintenance and equipment to branding, PR, apparel, moral and logistical support. I will be forever grateful to so many people for making this possible.

The Storms Before the Storms

Preparing for The World's Toughest Row was far from plain sailing. The cautionary words from others that the hardest part would be getting to the start line proved to be wise words.

We were fortunate to have been lent an R45 ocean rowing boat, Mrs Nelson. She is the matriarch of ocean rowing boats, the first of her kind to be built, with the number 1 on her hull. She'd done five successful crossings before us, including

David's, so she had considerable pedigree, which imbued us with faith in her ability to carry us safely across. However, she also bore the hallmarks of a boat that has seen a few storms. We were well matched in many ways, proudly wearing the scars we'd earned through life's storms.

And just as we needed some patching up at times, Mrs Nelson was in and out of minor injuries and occasional surgery during training. We'd hoped she might just need a cosmetic polish, but over the course of our training, everything we touched seemed to fall apart. The make-up job became more of a major overhaul – new batteries, a complete rewiring, new cabin doors, navigation and steering technology upgraded and replaced, new solar panels, new life raft – the list was endless. Whenever we thought we were nearly there with repairs, something else would rear its head. Fortunately, the race organisers, Atlantic Campaigns, made timely inspections to ensure each crew was on track to be ready to race, so we knew what had to be done by when.

Even so, we nearly missed our shipping slot because the final set of tweaks was more like major surgery than finishing touches. The relaxed weekend we'd planned in Burnham, showing our children the boat and meticulously checking and carefully packing all of our kit, turned into an after-work dash to Essex, packing everything we'd need for our crossing in the middle of a freezing night by the light of a couple of head torches, before retreating the same night to be back for work and the school run the next morning. When all else failed, humour was our saviour. The only way through it was to do it, and laughter is much more conducive to progress than tears. There was no time for methodical packing, so hula-hoops were crammed in alongside toilet rolls, yoga mats and explosive flares. There would be time to sort it out in La Gomera…

Our boat issues didn't end there. With less than a week to go before race day, we had our final inspection by the race safety team in La Gomera, an exercise in offloading every single piece of kit and equipment from the boat, laying it out in military fashion and checking our understanding of how to use everything. We almost passed with flying colours, save for tightening a loose bolt in the stern cabin. Pip grabbed the tools and set to work, but the bolt simply spun around. We called in one of the safety team to help, and, after a few more wiggles, the bolt came away in his hands, leaving an exposed hole right through the boat's hull. So with just days to go until we were due to cast off into 5,000 km of ocean, we had a hole right through our boat.

Leaning over the side of the boat, muttering profanities under my breath and with my heart in my mouth, I looked anxiously from Pip, who was wielding the sheared bolt in her hand, to the safety officers, desperately hoping they'd have a solution. We hadn't come this far to be halted in our tracks now.

News of the latest mishap to have befallen The Mothership spread through the boat park like wildfire, and soon enough, one by one, rowers arrived offering an array of spare bolts. Each time, a bolt of hope would raise our spirits, only to be crushed again when it didn't fit.

Unfortunately, as the oldest boat in the fleet, Mrs Nelson needed specialist parts, and the only place to source a new bolt was the original boat builders in the UK. It was time to call for help. Determined to find a solution, a few anxious phone calls later, we had a plan. One of the boat builder's team was due to fly out a few days later and would bring us the critical part we needed. It would delay our launch into the water, but we could breathe again.

The boat builder arrived, the hole was repaired and we eventually launched Mrs Nelson, to the collective relief of all concerned and applause from our fellow crews. We were several days later into the water than most boats, but we were there, and that's all that mattered at that point.

Challenges are sent to try us, and we can let them knock us down, drain us and defeat us. Or we can use them to grow stronger. As my fabulous friend Emma Henderson says, "Challenges don't define us, they refine us." We had many more than our fair share of challenges during training, but in their own way, they were all preparing us for the challenge of a lifetime that lay ahead. Life moves in mysterious ways, and while we often bored anyone who'd listen with the curveballs we faced, I think it was life's way of teaching us the lessons we needed to properly equip ourselves for the challenge of the mighty Atlantic Ocean. We'd been knocked down, picked ourselves up repeatedly, and made it to the start line full of relief, courage, resilience, determination and strength.

While Mrs Nelson went through many rounds of maintenance and repair, so did The Mothership crew. Rowing an ocean is not a decision to take lightly, particularly when you have dependents. It's not a decision you can take alone. Throughout our training, we had several changes to our crew as the reality of what we were taking on took hold or family circumstances changed. While Pip, Jo (a school mum friend of Pip) and I were in it from the start, we had to say goodbye to Sian, Laura and Paula during this time. And although they weren't part of the final crew, they all played their part in our journey. Each crew change posed a new challenge – to recruit someone who not only had the drive and determination to take on such a feat, but also a family network willing and able to plug the gap.

On top of that, they had to meet our recruitment requirements. As The Mothership, we'd limited our pool to mums, and they had to be the right fit with the rest of the crew. Team dynamics was an incredibly important consideration – the risk of team relationships imploding mid-Atlantic really doesn't bear thinking about, and 40+ days sharing a tiny boat with people you don't like isn't a prospect anyone wants to face.

Our final recruitment decision came just six months before the race started, when we were again reduced to a crew of three. This period was a critical time for us. Race rules state that each crew must complete 150 hours of rowing on the boat as a complete crew. We'd already completed our mandatory hours, but now reduced to three, we had to decide whether we tried to recruit a fourth and have to go back to square one and start our training hours over again, or continue forward as a three. Both options were viable, but both had their difficulties.

Recruiting a fourth crew member at this late stage in the day would not be easy; finding someone willing and able to drop normal life at short notice would be tricky, and then the logistics of fitting in all of the training, mandatory courses and mandatory hours on the boat would be tight for both the new member and existing crew. On the flip side, rowing as a three-person team was not what we'd signed up for. It would, in all likelihood, mean a slower crossing, more time away from our families, and a complete change in our shift patterns and routines. As a four, you never row alone; you always have company on deck – someone to share the highs and lows with, laugh and occasionally cry with, and keep you awake when your body screams for sleep. And the shift patterns of a four are reasonably straightforward – generally two hours on and two hours off, with two people rowing at a time. As a three, the shift pattern is a lot more complicated, and someone generally has to row on their own a lot of the time. We didn't want to do that if we didn't absolutely have to.

After discussions with Atlantic Campaigns, we gave ourselves a deadline and resolved to try and find a replacement by that point, but failing that, we'd go as a three. For once during our campaign, the heavens aligned. Enter Lebby, a great university friend of Jo's. As a mother, freelance journalist and Oxford Blue rower who had recently started rowing again, she had the freedom to take time out. Moreover, we knew Lebby, and Lebby knew what she was letting herself in for, having interviewed us as a crew for an article in *The Telegraph* just a few weeks earlier. We invited Lebby to join us for a weekend outing on Mrs Nelson, and 36 laughter-packed hours later, we were back to being a four – this time, the final four.

COVID, with its lockdowns, bubbles, tiers and social distancing rules, proved an interesting stakeholder during our two-year preparation, insisting on us frequently having to adapt our plans, put training outings on ice and work out new ways of doing things. Although we were lucky to have a boat throughout our preparation (some crews only have one season to train on their boat), COVID restrictions meant that opportunities to meet in person as a crew and train on the boat were few and far between, particularly during our first year of training. We'd spend hours coordinating four sets of family diaries to accommodate training outings, only to repeat the exercise when a new lockdown or bubble rules came into play.

In the same way that the working world switched to a virtual landscape as much as possible, so did we. Team meetings were held on Zoom, including a team-bonding black-tie dinner party, during which we sampled the freeze-dried rations we'd take on the boat. Where possible, training courses switched to online learning, making our lives easier and reducing the time we'd travel and be away from home. We each managed to cobble together enough physical training equipment to do our physical training from home and made reasonable progress.

A Steep Learning Curve

The most significant impact was on our ability to train on the water, which is a critical part of preparation. We'd all rowed before to at least a reasonable level, either at school, university or both. But, as we were to discover, ocean rowing is a somewhat different kettle of fish from river rowing. They both involve boats, oars and seats, but that's about where the similarities end.

We were four intrepid, independent-spirited women who knew how to row and liked to think we were capable and intelligent, so we decided we could probably work out how to launch our boat, Mrs Nelson, and take her for a paddle. Around six months after deciding to enter the race, one weekend in early October, we finally found a window in the COVID restrictions to meet in Essex for our first outing. At the time, we thought it was a reasonably successful first outing, and perhaps in some ways it was, if you account for all the lessons we learned. However, in retrospect, it's a miracle we made it into the water afloat, let alone back out again, because we didn't have a clue what we were doing. We were blissfully ignorant of how much we didn't know.

Gathering in the misty October morning, with the sun battling to break through, there was a palpable excitement in the air – the expectation of an adventure about to begin. We were bubbling with anticipation, chattering like schoolgirls on the first day of term. Brimming with energy and the confidence that comes with naivety, we set to work preparing Mrs Nelson for the short tow to the marina.

None of us had ever towed anything before, or knew how to hitch a trailer to a car, but, undeterred, we had a go and weaved our way cautiously along the lanes the short distance to the marina. Towing forwards was one thing – reversing a trailer down a slipway to launch the boat was another matter. With our confidence quickly evaporating but determination keeping us going, it took many attempts, an awfully long time, a damaged rudder and many bemused onlookers before we got even remotely close to launching Mrs Nelson. The slipway lived up to its name, resulting in a heart-stopping moment when the car lost its grip, wheels angrily spinning and engine screaming in protest, and we feared it might also be launched. But somehow we managed it, got all four of us onboard, manoeuvred safely around the marina's many more conventional and expensive-looking boats and breathed a sigh of relief as we turned into the wide open river for a paddle.

With smug and smiling faces, we congratulated ourselves on a job not exactly well done, but done anyway, and settled into a rowing rhythm.

We decided to head downstream and soon left the marina behind us. We'd escaped the mayhem of family life, we were finally doing ocean rowing – albeit on a river – and, to top it off, we'd come prepared with a flask of freshly brewed black coffee and iced buns. Leaning against the doorway of the bow cabin, sipping thermos coffee and munching contentedly on a bun, listening to the rhythmic sound of the oars breaking the water and feeling the tug of the boat, I thought, "Life doesn't get much better than this." It was bliss after the confinement of lockdown and the pandemonium and frustration of home schooling. And after talking about ocean rowing for six months, it was a relief to finally do it. It felt like a giant leap forward in our journey.

We made excellent progress down the river and, after a couple of hours, decided to turn around and head back up, possibly even venturing out into the sea. The return leg proved to be trickier. Tides had been with us on the outbound leg, and they were most definitely against us on the way back. The boat felt heavy in the water, and each stroke of the oar was like weightlifting. The oars became increasingly painful to handle as our hands grew tender and inflamed with the constant friction of feathering (twisting the oar to bring the spoon parallel with the water while you prepare to take a stroke). We rowed for hours, making little progress. What's more, we struggled to keep the boat in a straight line or balanced, and had to make many adjustments to our steering.

After battling on for some time and feeling a little less pleased with ourselves, a paddleboarder appeared alongside, offering to help. We clearly looked like we needed some help. Fortunately for us, the paddleboarder was the electrician from the boat builders, so he knew Mrs Nelson and knew more than we did about ocean rowing boats. He suggested we use our centreboard to help keep the boat straight. "What's that?" was our baffled response. A quick lesson in centreboards followed, and although it sounded like the answer to some of our struggles, it transpired that ours was not working – a job for the rapidly growing to-do list.

Eventually we made it back to the marina and, against the odds, managed to get Mrs Nelson out of the water and back onto the relative safety of her trailer – not without a few words from the marina manager, who had witnessed the shenanigans earlier in the morning and was on standby for our return. We were not at all versed in marina etiquette and had failed to book or pay for our launch, but a few friendly words later and fees paid, we promised to try harder next time, and he sent us on our way.

Outing one: done. It would be a stretch to call it a roaring success, but we made it back in one piece and learnt a lot. The journey home was more reflective than the outward journey, having realised that our earlier confidence was premature.

Ocean rowing was quite different from river rowing, and if the state of our hands was anything to go by, we had a lot of conditioning to do before we'd be anywhere near ready to cross the Atlantic.

Some time later, when Pip was debriefing David on the trip and showing him her blistered hands, we realised the error of our ways. Feathering is not a technique used in ocean rowing – no endless turning of the clunky oars and the friction of the wooden handle in your hands. The lightbulb moment was a relief because we'd all wondered how on earth our hands and wrists would cope with weeks and weeks of that, but it was probably also the wake-up call we needed. If we got that wrong, what else didn't we know? We realised that we needed to know what we didn't know. We needed to ask people to help us and find people who knew more about ocean rowing than we did. "Find an ocean-rowing coach" was added to the top of the to-do list.

Ocean rowing is a small world, and it didn't take us long to find "Rowing Roy" – Duncan – and persuade him to take us on. If our first outing had exposed a few cracks in our ocean-rowing armoury, then our first weekend spent with Duncan reduced our armoury to splinters on the ground. It was an exposé on how much we didn't know and had to learn. But we were in excellent hands with Duncan. We had a plan, and we knew we could learn.

The first day with Duncan was spent getting to know the boat, running through the equipment and how everything worked, and learning the theory of how to row an ocean rowing boat. The second day, we planned an outing in Mrs Nelson, putting some of the theory into practice. But as time passed, we realised quite how much essential equipment we were missing and how ill-prepared we had been for our first outing.

Duncan: "Where are your safety harnesses?"

Me: "What are they?" (It turns out they are the number one safety rule of ocean rowing – you must be attached to the boat at all times.)

Duncan: "Where's your radio?"

We looked at one another. "I don't think we have one?" Pip offered.

Duncan: "Where's your water to stabilise the boat?"

We had quizzical, slightly embarrassed expressions on our faces. It would explain why we spent our first outing bobbing around, tipping from one side to the other.

Each question, with the lack of satisfactory answer, revealed another chink in our armoury.

But what we did have in spades was enthusiasm, a willingness to learn and work hard. Oh, and two bags for life full of M&S snacks. We used these to placate Duncan, and I like to think we still hold the crown for the best rowing snacks.

It was a lesson in managing expectations. We'd set a pretty low bar, but at least Duncan knew what he had to contend with. I'm sure he wondered whether we'd all bitten off more than we could chew at this point, and it would have been understandable if he'd chosen to run for the hills. But Duncan's an ocean rower – taking on challenges comes with the territory – and he rose to the challenge, eyes wide open. Perhaps he also saw something in the relentless determination and blind positivity of these four women that gave him some hope.

We knew how much we didn't know and took every opportunity we could to learn. Our preparation didn't get any easier, and we continued to face challenges, make mistakes and learn. But that's all part of the process. Training is learning exactly when to make mistakes, so you learn how not to do that again when it really counts.

One of the idiosyncrasies of training to row the Atlantic is that many of the skills you need to learn for training are not skills you're likely to need to row an ocean. Navigating the coastal waters of the UK came with the challenges of scores of other boats, hazards to avoid, anchorage and tides, to name a few. Those are things you're unlikely to encounter during an

Atlantic row. An anchor isn't going to be much help when you're in 5 km depth of water; on the whole, you're unlikely to come even remotely close to any other boats or fixed hazards, and tides aren't a consideration. But all challenges help build your resilience and ability to adapt, even if the specific challenge isn't something you'll find in the race.

One particularly low point was during a long, cold weekend row, when we were based out of Gosport Marina. We'd had an eventful night, managing very little sleep while we tried to avoid being marooned in marshland, and mental and physical resources were depleted. But we pressed on and headed out of Portsmouth Harbour into the open sea to clock up a few more hours and miles. Unfortunately, lots of other boats had chosen to head in or out of the harbour at the same time, and while the tides were against us and the waves were causing mayhem, we found ourselves playing chicken with two approaching ferries. We were clearly the underdogs in this contest and didn't fancy our chances.

As we hauled on the oars, desperately trying to get some purchase and turn the boat, I suddenly felt very small and insignificant. The waves meant we struggled to get any traction with either our oars or the steering, and, with each ineffective stroke, the ferries both loomed larger. The sound of their engines grew louder, drowning out our voices, and we bobbed precariously in the turbulent waves. I looked from left to right with alarm as the water rose around and above us, gritting my teeth and bracing myself for an imminent soaking – or worse.

Seeing no way out of this predicament, we concluded it was time to use our new radio. With the reassurance of help on the way and assistance from some favourable waves, we manoeuvred ourselves out of immediate danger, and minutes later, a police rescue boat pulled up alongside. With a mixture of relief and wounded pride, we relinquished control of Mrs Nelson and reluctantly agreed to be towed back into the marina, tails well and truly tucked between our legs.

When we were safely tied up on the jetty, one of the policemen remarked that we looked exhausted and should probably call it a day. Jo's response still makes me smile: "No, we're mums. This is what we always look like."

At that moment, we had a decision to make: Do we abandon our outing to lick our wounds, or reset and start again? We chose the latter. We knew we'd made an error of judgment trying to head out to sea at that time, with the conditions we faced, but we'd learned a lesson. We planned a different, more gentle route down the river that would help us regain confidence and, importantly, keep us moving forward. Challenges may knock you down, but the important thing is learning to pick yourself up, reset and keep going. Be mindful of the experience and what it's taught you, and be not afraid to carry on.

Had we abandoned our outings each time we came up against a challenge, we would never have completed our mandatory hours or made it to the start line. Because our training years were punctuated by a litany of mishaps and misadventures – sometimes, but not always, of our own making. A few incidents in particular stand out in my mind:

> Hitting our top training speed in the dead of night on a fast-flowing current. The initial glee was soon replaced with dread as we realised we couldn't stop and were careering into a stretch of river densely populated with moored and unlit boats.

> Pip commenting on how far out from the shore some people seemed to be standing, swiftly followed by being grounded on a south coast sandbank until the tide turned.

> Not noticing that we'd parted company with a mooring buoy and were about to hit the bank.

> "Petrol forecourt gate." The national petrol shortage nearly caused us to miss our shipping slot. Lebby saved the day by indignantly and loudly confronting outraged customers on the forecourt as I hid behind the car door, surreptitiously filling can after can.

> Bodywork (our own) falling into disrepair – broken wrist, neck operation, torn muscles, cancer scare.

What doesn't kill you makes you stronger. When I look back on the early days of our training, I realise the extent of the oceans we crossed just to get to the start line. I barely recognise now the hapless crew that we were. But what we lacked in practical ocean-rowing skills and ability, we made up for in mental ability, mindset and resilience. Decades of working, parenting and generally surviving the knocks of life had given us an invaluable foundation that no textbook or coach could teach us. Age was our advantage. We wore it and used it with pride.

Chapter 5
Hanging in the Balance

My alarm sounded, and it felt like the dead of night. I lay there for a moment, staring into the darkness to get my bearings, then gathered my thoughts. It was 29 November 2021, and my last night at home before flying out with Lebby, Jo and Pip to take our place on the start line of The World's Toughest Row. I had already packed my bags, given the children my leaving gifts and said my goodbyes to them. I was leaving at 6 am, so I didn't want to wake them from their slumber.

Before we went to sleep, Paul had turned to me and said how unexpectedly sad he felt. I think it was intended as a compliment. Everyone's concern had been focused on how the children would cope without Mummy, easing the emotional burden for them, but they weren't the only ones being left behind. It was quite something to see your life partner – the person you love most in the world – pack their bags and leave for the adventure of a lifetime, but one that carried inherent risk. Paul had been a tower of strength and joy for the children, but he would miss me, too.

I crept out of bed, trying not to wake Paul, had a quick shower, got dressed and was ready to leave. As I was about to head down the stairs, Ben, our six-year-old middle son, appeared from his bedroom. He wanted to say goodbye again. I lifted him up and held him tight. I told him I loved him, to look after his brother and sister and to be good for Daddy. He was an unusually perceptive little fellow, and he asked me to go and say goodbye to Sam, our eldest, saying, "He'd want you to wake him and say goodbye, Mummy." That was when I crumbled, realising how much this was weighing on their little minds, filling their thoughts, waking them from their sleep. I hugged Paul and the boys again through teary eyes, opened the front door and stepped out into the night to begin the final leg of our journey to the start line.

Jo, Pip, Lebby and I convened at Heathrow, meeting at the departure gates, laden with rucksacks stuffed with an unusual array of apparel. With the exception of my parents, our families weren't coming out to La Gomera to see us off, so anything that wasn't coming on Mrs Nelson with us had to be kept to the bare miniMum.

We were full of excitement and disbelief that the moment had finally arrived. There were still a few tears as we recounted snippets of our emotional farewells, but it was onwards with the task at hand – getting ourselves to La Gomera to begin our final preparations and countdown to the race start. Besides Jo, who was suffering the effects of a nasty cold, we were bouncing with energy and raring to go, like pop bottles ready to explode.

The journey passed smoothly. We were delighted to see another couple of crews on the flight and bonded immediately over the shared adventure that lay ahead.

A COVID Curve Ball

La Gomera was reached by ferry from Tenerife, and it was as we sat on a bench at the La Gomera ferry terminal, waiting for a taxi, that Jo commented, "I can't taste anything and I can't smell anything." The telltale symptoms of COVID. Those words sent a shiver down my spine. We looked at each other nervously, desperately hoping that our worst nightmare might not be about to come true. It was November 2021 when a positive COVID test meant self-isolation, and the risk of transmission was high. I shuffled along the bench a little – a futile attempt to put some distance between me and possible COVID infection.

Abandoning the wait for a taxi, we struggled up the steep streets of San Sebastián with our heavy bags, Jo becoming increasingly breathless with the effort. Finally arriving at our apartment, we settled Jo into a mercifully self-contained room, separated from the rest of the apartment by two heavy doors, and set out into town in search of a pharmacy.

Having procured COVID tests, vitamins, antiviral spray, protective gloves and masks, we nervously returned to the apartment and posted a test through Jo's door. Within minutes, she confirmed what we'd feared: a positive test. Our bubble of excitement and anticipation was well and truly burst, our dreams and hopes crumbling around us.

It was time to face our biggest challenge yet – the mental torture of not knowing if we'd get to race after pouring our hearts and souls into the campaign for the best part of two years. What would happen if one of the remaining three tested positive in the next few days? What if Jo was too sick to race? What if we weren't allowed out to prepare the boat or take part in the race briefings? So many what-if scenarios were flying around our heads – a blur of questions and possibilities. Having travelled out together, posing for group selfies and sharing food for nearly 12 hours, the chance of one of us not also testing positive over the following days seemed remote.

We had 13 days before the race started – just enough time for Jo to recover, get through quarantine and make it to the start line. But if anyone else tested positive in the next few days, we'd have run out of time. It would have meant an agonising, heart-wrenching decision: Would we go as a three (and which three would it be?), would we not go at all or postpone until another year?

The following few days were torturous, not least for Jo, who was quarantined inside a room with hardly any home comforts and full-blown COVID. She faced the fear that she might not be well enough to race, the fear we all shared that she might not be the only one of us to go down with COVID, and the deep sense of isolation as the rest of the fleet carried on with their final preparations.

Pip, Lebby and I went through the nerve-racking daily routine of waking up, lying in bed swallowing, trying to determine if we had normal dry morning throat or COVID throat, if our grogginess was just the hangover of sleep or something more sinister, then gathering around the dining room table for synchronised COVID testing. The anguish of the 15-minute wait while we hardly dared to look at the little white sticks, followed by the high-fiving, the temporary relief and then cracking on with the endless list of jobs we needed to do before being ready to race. To say it was a test of nerves would be an understatement, but we found respite in comedy and community.

I had no recollection of exactly what we laughed about, but I remembered sitting around the table, tears rolling down our faces, finding humour in the farcical predicament we were in. There was also a significant amount of time doomscrolling to try to work out how likely we were to get COVID, whether there were any magic foods or supplements we could take to fend it off (we were willing to throw money at the problem), when we'd be most likely to test positive, and therefore when we could start to breathe again.

While Jo battled with COVID – with a wracking cough, fever, headache and aching limbs – we took every precaution we could think of to protect ourselves from infection. When called on to deliver food supplies to Jo, Lebby went the extra mile and decked herself out in elbow-length gloves, a full mask and a hat, instructing Jo to stay well back as she hastily delivered one tray and collected another. The rigmarole that followed was equally comical, with everything that could be destroyed torn up and tossed out, all crockery diligently disinfected and every inch of available skin scrubbed until it was an angry pink.

After a week or so, Jo's symptoms gradually abated, and her general malaise was replaced by frustration at not being able to experience the pre-race build-up or be involved in the final preparations, alongside an eagerness to escape confinement and embed herself in fleet life.

Community Over Competition

Miraculously, Lebby, Pip and I seemed to have dodged the COVID bullet, and after a few days, we finally allowed ourselves to believe that we would all be able to take our places on the start line. Renamed "COVID Crew," we were integrated into the rest of the fleet, welcomed by a round of applause on our first appearance in the race tent. Although we did our best to keep our distance, desperately not wanting to pass anything on, it was wonderful to finally meet the other crews and share this unique experience with them. We were a kinship – people from all walks of life and corners of the world, brought together by the same dream: to row, unaided, 3,000 miles across the inhospitable Atlantic Ocean, and achieve something that very few people had ever done.

Although we were competitors, the overriding spirit was one of community – every crew genuinely willing each other on and doing everything possible to ensure the fleet's success. I had rarely experienced such a powerful demonstration of collective generosity, support and care for people who, until days earlier, were strangers. As one rower put it, we were all there because we said, "I can, and I will."

With ground to make up after COVID interrupted play, other crews came to our rescue, offering help with packing, unpacking, last-minute maintenance and kit inspections. There was a flourishing black market in missing or excess kits; rowers would sidle up to other crews, offering surplus supplies in exchange for a vital missing item. We were the grateful recipients of many treasured things – from a flare (turned out to be very useful) and solar shower (useless, if you're considering one), to a BGAN (a very expensive communication device to generate an internet connection via satellites) and reflective bubble wrap to keep the sun out of the cabins.

Arguably our finest trade – certainly for Jo and me, who ate most of it – was a chef-produced dehydrated Christmas dinner for four, complete with cranberry sauce and pigs-in-blankets, in exchange for a chunk of my homemade Christmas cake. We were cock-a-hoop bringing that little gem back to Mrs Nelson. It became a carrot dangling in front of us for the first two weeks of rowing – something to mark Christmas Day as a little different to the other 39 days on board.

Those final days of preparation passed in a haze of activity: last-minute packing, race briefings, medical checks, learning how to use our new communications devices, downloading playlists, media interviews, finding and fixing the hole in our boat, orientation rows – the list went on. As race day approached, the ferry terminal brought a constant stream of crew friends and family, anxiously awaiting the final farewells. San Sebastián came alive as restaurants played host to family dinners, and the buzz of expectation filled the air.

Just as the rowers had bonded in the previous days, the arriving supporters bonded over their experience of being the ones left behind – the bizarre mix of excitement, anticipation, fear, dread and pride. The row was not just a test of endurance for the rowers; the supporters or "dot watchers" had their own unique endurance event ahead of them: 3,000 miles of anxiously waiting for the race app's four-hourly position updates, and more sporadic contact from the rowers themselves.

Mum and Dad arrived a couple of days before race day, and their presence was a joy and welcome distraction for us all. They adopted the role of honorary Mothership parents, providing love, support and a calming influence not just for Pip and me, but also for Lebby and Jo.

When you're about to embark on an adventure into the unknown, where anything could happen and your vulnerability against the raw force of nature is exposed, there is something incredibly stabilising, grounding, reassuring and comforting about having your parents close. Your inner child breathes a sigh of relief – a feeling of safety washing over you – because parents make everything okay. As a parent myself, I now know that our instinct to parent and protect never leaves us, and our own yearning to feel safe and protected never leaves us either.

Wild horses wouldn't have stopped Mum and Dad from coming out to see us start and be there to give us one final, gripping hug on race day. But cancer made it more of a challenge for Dad than I think we realised at the time. Dad had been diagnosed with stage 4 kidney cancer in 2018 and, after recuperating from surgery to remove his kidney, had enjoyed an extended period of relatively good health, with the secondary tumours kept in check by various treatments. Dad was incredibly positive throughout his cancer journey –

determined to outwit the unwelcome invader and maintain a belief that where there is life, there is hope. Despite his terminal diagnosis, I wanted to believe he could beat it, and his long period of wellness had probably lulled me into false hope. But seeing Dad in La Gomera, outside his home environment, it was clear that cancer's grip was tightening.

The streets of San Sebastián are not for the faint-hearted, and steep roads and steps led up the hill to our apartment. We couldn't fail to notice how he struggled with the walk, stopping frequently to catch his breath, and it was heartbreaking to see how his health had deteriorated. But still we had hope, because he'd had dips before and had responded to treatment, so surely he could do that again.

As we counted down the days to the race start, I waited for the nerves to take hold. I kept expecting to wake up one morning and feel the fear hit me like a freight train – to be paralysed by what lay ahead, by what I was about to take on. When I first heard about the race, I'd been terrified of the prospect of being in a tiny boat in massive waves, and I thought the fear would return as the start drew nearer. But the countdown continued, and the fear stayed away. Even on race day itself, there were no nerves. I often reflected on why that was and put it down to our rigorous preparation.

Our training had been peppered with challenges we'd battled hard to overcome. We'd known adversity and conquered it. We'd fought to get ourselves to this point – even through the last-ditch attempt by COVID to scupper our plans – and I truly believed this preparation had served us well. Through nearly two years of training, we gradually adjusted to the idea of what we were taking on. We had scenario-planned for every eventuality we could, including expecting the unexpected.

We'd visualised 40-foot waves. We'd run through the capsize drill. We'd been on a sea survival course where we learned about the 3,001 ways to die at sea in an ocean rowing boat. We were expecting to face significant challenges and mentally tough times. Mentally and physically, we were ready for anything. They say you should train hard to fight easy – and while I would never describe the race as easy, the training was undoubtedly hard. The preparation had helped me embrace that fear, use it as fuel to channel into my training and see it as a positive. Without that fear, would I have felt as ready? I doubted it.

A cloud of anticipation hung over the streets of San Sebastián the evening before the race start. The restaurants were full of families gathered together one final time before saying goodbye to their loved ones. Where, a few days earlier, crews dined, laughed and chatted together, that evening was reserved for families. I don't think anyone knew whether to celebrate or commiserate – whether to laugh, cry or perhaps both. It was a strange cocktail of anticipation, excitement, adrenaline and nerves. Literally and metaphorically, it felt like the calm before the storm – an evening of waiting for the inevitable. Waiting for the last embrace, and finally beginning what we'd set out to do such a long time ago.

Returning to our apartment that evening, we set to work finishing our preparations – each of us lost in our own thoughts as we ticked off the items in our boat bags one final time and packed everything else away to return home with Mum and Dad.

Mum appeared in my room while I was packing and gave me two laminated cards. On one, she'd printed a meditation, and on the other, a passage from the Bible. We hugged as she told me she loved me and to look after each other. She'd obviously spent a long time thinking about the passages to give us, and the words were powerful and comforting.

They were a reminder that someone was looking out for us, a reminder to be brave and strong. Dad is normally the one for emotive words, speeches and gestures, and I've lost count of the number of times he'd made himself and others cry with his heart-on-sleeve approach, while Mum would smile on, indulging Dad's outpouring of emotion. So this gesture from Mum spoke volumes. I'd managed to hold it together until this point, but those words, and what they represented, brought me to tears. At that moment, I truly appreciated what it must have felt like for Mum and Dad to watch their two daughters embark on such an extreme adventure. They must have felt such pride, love and support for what we were doing – and such heart-wrenching fear for what might lie ahead for us.

I carefully packed those cards away, knowing they would comfort and inspire me during the adventure that was about to unfold.

>An excerpt from A Meditation by Frances J Roberts:

>"Move on steadily,
>and know that the waters that carry you
>are the waters of My love and My kindness,
>and I will keep you on the right course."

Chapter 6
Losing Sight of Land

From Chaos to Calm: The Final Hours on Dry Land

Race day dawned, and we were still not ready. I'd imagined a relaxed start – luxuriating in my last hot shower, a final breakfast together, maybe even a bit of quiet yoga to settle our nerves before joining the other crews in the race tent. But the reality was far removed from that zen experience I'd conjured up.

Instead, we were tearing around the apartment, throwing kits into bags in a haphazard fashion, emptying cupboards of leftover provisions, making endless trips to the bins with mounds of rubbish, making up sandwiches for the first few meals, boiling water to save us a job in the first 24 hours and hailing a taxi to take Mum and Dad to their hotel. The rush spared us a long, drawn-out and emotional farewell with my parents, and I was relieved to have had a million and one things to distract me from that goodbye. We grabbed our boat bags and hurried to the race tent at an anxious trot. We made a breathless and sweaty entrance, but we were there, and after all of the hurdles and metaphorical oceans we'd crossed to get there, that was all that mattered.

The atmosphere in the tent that morning was electric. For everyone, this was the culmination of years of training, trials and tribulations, a day that many wondered would ever come. Yet here we all were, because we said, "I can, and I will."

Sitting alongside Pip, Jo and Lebby, it was hard not to get swept up in the emotion of the occasion. Ripples of excitement coursed through the tent as crews exchanged final encouraging words, last-minute advice or humorous anecdotes from the final farewells. It was a time of collective anticipation as we sat on the brink of our journey into the unknown, interspersed with moments of personal reflection. My broad smile was occasionally brought in check by sudden, unexpected swells of emotion. I raised my eyes to the roof of the briefing tent, breathing deeply and blinking my brimming eyes to settle myself.

After a few brief but rousing words from the race team, like warriors unleashed for war, we left the race tent and made our way into the marina for the final time. The route to the marina was unusually busy, filled with a throng of rowers, family and other supporters. Weaving our way through the crowds, we passed tearful embrace after tearful embrace – rowers in a hurry to get to their boats, loved ones clinging on to extend the final moments. As the secure gate into the lower pontoon closed behind us, it was time to switch our focus from the families we were leaving to the task ahead. We followed the procession of rowers to take our places on the waiting boats.

The walkway around the marina was lined with supporters, two or three deep, soaking in the extraordinary atmosphere of race day. Crews busied themselves on their boats, securing the final bits of luggage and equipment, checking and double-checking that the tech was working. Keeping busy was a diversion tactic, something to fill the remaining minutes before the start.

I'd expected to feel the nerves biting – the butterflies and stomach-turning sensation you get when you're about to do something that scares you. But in contrast to the cacophony of sounds and hum of activity around us, I felt a strange sense of calmness.

I occupied myself putting away the few personal possessions I'd brought (there's no room for luxuries), stowing Mum's laminated passages in a pocket in the cabin where I could easily access them. I reflected on how far we'd come and the oceans we'd crossed to reach this point. I was excited and intrigued about what we were about to do, but the overriding emotions were relief and gratitude. Relief that we'd made it through so many challenges, that all four of us had made it to the start line and were lining up together to do what we'd been planning for such a long time. And gratitude, gratitude that Covid hadn't stolen this opportunity, gratitude to all those people who had supported us to get this far and gratitude to be one of the very few people who had the privilege of experiencing something so extraordinary.

Crews were starting in reverse number order from 37, three minutes apart, with the larger crews first and finishing with the fearless solo rowers. We were boat 32, so we had a few minutes to wait while the first boats departed. Nothing could have prepared us for the experience of the race start. It was truly unforgettable.

As each boat was released from its mooring by the race safety officers and the crew took its first tentative strokes through the calm water of the marina, the other crews stood in their boats, cheering and whooping in solidarity, with the backdrop of hundreds of supporters on the upper pontoon doing the same. It was a spontaneous celebration and acknowledgement of the whole fleet's collective determination, resilience and courage – a show of mutual respect and admiration for what we'd all been through and what we were about to embark on. Looking along the line of boats to our right, we watched the gaps appear, one by one, like dominoes, as we said farewell to competitors and now friends.

And then it was our turn.

3,000 Miles to Row

The race officials untied our mooring lines as Ian Couch held on to our boat and started the countdown. The race camera crew hovered on the pontoon, capturing the moment of our departure. One minute. Some final words of advice: "Stay safe, ladies, and see you in Antigua." Thirty seconds. A final look up to Mum and Dad, a smile and a wave. Ten seconds. I picked up my oar handles and felt Mrs Nelson move away from the pontoon as Ian gently pushed us off at 11.10 am on 12 December 2021. Sitting in the bow seat, I was the first to get my oars clear, and I came forward on the slide, raised my hands to feel the oars connect with the water, and took the first of around 1.5 million oar strokes to Antigua.

Lebby and Pip soon joined in, and we cautiously manoeuvred our way through the waiting boats and the marina, to the incredible cheers and shouts from the other crews and supporters. As we looked around, it was hard to take in what was happening – all these people cheering for us, as we had cheered for those who'd left before us – and the sense of being part of a truly unique and special community was palpable.

With Jo at the helm, we turned the corner into the marina entrance and, with a hoot of a horn, crossed the start line of the World's Toughest Row. The last voice I heard as we pulled away from the crowds was Duncan, our ocean rowing coach, who'd come out to La Gomera like a proud dad to see his crews start. And that was it. We were on our way and, in all likelihood, wouldn't see another soul until we arrived in Antigua.

We were a bundle of excitement and chatter as we pulled away from La Gomera. We couldn't believe what we'd just experienced – the thrill, joy and pride to be part of something so incredible was something we all felt, and those feelings carried us through for a long, long time.

Amidst the chatter, Jo got to work tidying away fenders, ropes and equipment that we wouldn't need again until we reached land on the other side. Pip, Lebby and I put in the first shift on the oars and settled into a steady rhythm. At that stage, there was still lots to see around us – a few sailing boats, land alongside, and a little stream of tiny ocean rowing boats, all charting a slightly different course out of the marina and into the open sea. It was impossible to identify the different boats, but we tried nonetheless, and also tried to work out whether we were catching up or being caught. Soon enough, the other crews became tiny dots or disappeared entirely from view, and we were on our own. It was the four of us, Mrs Nelson and the vast Atlantic Ocean.

We rowed "three up" until sunset, each rowing for 90 minutes, followed by a 30-minute break to fuel and rest before starting again. This routine meant we could make some good distance quickly, leveraging the time when we weren't feeling the effects of lack of sleep or seasickness. At sunset, we reverted to our standard pattern of two hours "on," two hours "off," with two people rowing and two people resting. Lebby and I, sharing the bow cabin and bow seat, rotated on the odd hours, while Pip and Jo, sharing the stern cabin and the middle seat, rotated on the even hours. That meant we got to row with one person for an hour, then another for the second hour. That was important, not just because it meant a change in conversation and entertainment, but also because it meant that every hour, at least, something was happening to break up the monotony of the shift and something to mark the halfway point. Particularly during the night shifts, that change of crew halfway through was a morale boost. Knowing you'd be the next to clamber back into the comfort of the cabin to snatch a few precious minutes' sleep gave me the motivation to push on through the second hour.

During that first day, before fatigue set in, it was difficult to sleep during off shifts. So I sat in the cabin, ate some food, and tried to absorb the experience of the last few hours. Thirty minutes passed very quickly, and soon enough I was back on the oars and relieved to be on deck in the fresh air again. Seasickness was starting to creep in, but fortunately for me, only when confined in the cabin. Pip, however, didn't fare so well and, pretty soon, she felt the effects and would stop mid-shift to vomit over the side. Her seasickness continued for the next two days. As the person who sat behind her for much of the time – and as her sister – it was awful to see, but there was no option but to keep going. We knew that seasickness was likely, and we also knew it could continue for a long time.

It wasn't a reason to stop, because that would put more pressure on everyone else. It was simply something you had to tolerate and get through for as long as it continued. With the sea state being relatively calm, we were lucky to get away lightly with sickness – a little nausea for Jo, Lebby and me, and a couple of days of feeling rotten for Pip – but she battled through valiantly, and soon enough was out the other side.

Finding Our Sea Legs

Our propensity to negotiate the row safely, happily and quickly hinged on our ability to adapt to the new world around us. Those first few hours and days were an exercise in learning how to live at sea in a tiny rowing boat. We had to learn how to mentally adapt and figure out how to move safely around the boat, including the basic daily functions of sleeping, eating, toileting and hygiene. When you stood on the start line in La Gomera and looked out to sea, you knew that Antigua was far beyond the horizon.

Three thousand miles is an unfathomable distance to row and, unlike most races, you could only make an educated and hopeful guess at how long it would take. You might have set a goal – in our case, it was under 45 days – but there was so much out of your control, and so much unknown, that it was finger in the air at best. You had to be mentally prepared to be out there, rowing, for as long as it took to arrive in Antigua.

That could be 35 days, 40 days, 50 days, or even 60 days. Some solo rowers may be out there for 100+ days.

If you focused solely on the finish line and the 3,000 miles you had to row, you'd quickly become demoralised by the lack of progress, the imperceptible dents you made each day into the miles you needed to cross. So the only way to approach it was to break it down into more palatable milestones, smaller goals you could realistically envisage reaching.

The start of the race was not about rowing to Antigua, but about the first milestones on the long journey that would eventually take us there. The first night on board was a significant step. Nights could be tough when you were tired, maybe scared, and often left with your thoughts. You had to adapt to sleeping efficiently and get used to a routine that was alien to most. There were no home comforts in an ocean rowing boat – just a thin foam mattress in a tiny, hot cabin, the same spot you sat in, ate in and relaxed in. The same spot where your cabin buddy did all those things, too.

A boat that tipped and rolled, sometimes gently, sometimes with angry violence; unfamiliar sounds all around as the waves crashed against the boat and the oars clunked rhythmically from the deck. No sooner were you asleep than your alarm sounded to rouse you for your next shift. Ninety minutes was the maximum time you'd spend asleep for the duration of the row. Everything in your body screamed sleep, yet you had to fight the urge to lie back down while you pulled on some clothes and clambered out of the tiny cabin door into the darkness to start a two-hour slog on the oars. Your ability to adapt to that routine and do it religiously for the row determined your success.

Although we'd spent several nights on board Mrs Nelson during our training around the UK coastline, it was only when you experienced your first full night on the Atlantic and emerged for your shift the following morning that you felt like a bona fide ocean rower. I remember the feeling of pride and accomplishment, climbing out of my cabin for my first shift of day two, having ticked off the first full night on board. And I hadn't just endured it – I'd enjoyed it.

The first full day was also significant because it was when you started cementing your routines and performing the daily tasks that would be critical to the crossing. Some tasks were different for each of us. I was the chief water boiler and maker, so I had to find the best way to boil water in a rocking boat without scalding myself, and I became a whizz in that particular extreme sport. We'd started the race with a supply of bottled water, but on day two, we had to start the daily routine of desalinating water to make our drinking water.

This process involved a tense few seconds while you waited for the all-important clunk from the water maker, then the spurt of waste water, signalling all was well and you could breathe once more. Lebby and I, responsible for all things water, shared the daily relief of hearing the water maker doing what it should. It was one of the essential pieces of equipment on the boat, which, if it failed, could mean the end of your race.

After a couple of days, we'd settled well into the rhythm of life at sea, enjoying this new experience and the unusual sense of freedom it offered. For the first few nights, you could still see the occasional navigation lights of other ocean rowing boats somewhere in the distance, but by day, there was no sign of anyone else. You were also losing sight of land. It was a significant moment when you looked around and all you could see was 360 degrees of blue – nothing to break up the horizon, whichever way you looked. Suddenly, you became aware of your insignificance on this vast planet that we inhabit, and that you were at the mercy of the might and power of Mother Nature that surrounds us. Losing sight of land could be overwhelming and was terrifying for many, but to me, it felt like freedom.

I was in awe of our incredible environment, intrigued by the journey ahead and at peace with whatever Mother Nature decided to serve us.

Chapter 7
Boat Life

Eat, Sleep, Row, Repeat

That's the usual routine for an ocean rower. After the initial excitement of the start and establishing our standard "two on, two off" shift pattern, we quickly settled into our new routine.

Ocean rowing life was refreshingly simple, in contrast to our less-than-ideal, pre-race build-up and the hectic, sometimes chaotic nature of normal life as a working parent. We'd done all the hard work to get to the start line, coordinating the multiple strands of our campaign alongside family and working life, and now all we had to do was eat, sleep, row, repeat.

It sounds simple, but of course, there's more to it than that.

The two-hour "sleep" shift is when you also have to make time for any other tasks that need to be done. Nothing is straightforward or quick on a boat tipping and rolling unpredictably in the waves, especially when you have to do everything while tethered to it by a two-metre strap.

During the first couple of days, we had to find our sea legs and become adept at travelling up and down the length of the deck. As a resident of the bow cabin, safely traversing the boat as quickly as possible to minimise disruption to the rowers and minimise your risk of flying overboard was paramount. The kitchen, bathroom and laundry all vied for positions in the admin area, which was the empty third rowing position at the opposite end of the boat in front of the stern cabin. Lebby, my cabin buddy, and I had to pick our way along the boat's length with any kit we needed, trying not to get tangled up in the tethers of the other rowers.

Cautious and clumsy at first, we anxiously scanned the horizon for oncoming waves that might slow us down. Every successful trip felt like a small victory in a long battle – each one worth celebrating. The empty third seat was a sanctuary of safety, somewhere we could breathe a small sigh of relief after the mini-adrenaline rush of the journey before carrying out our "admin" and bracing ourselves for the return leg. Soon, though, I was delighted to find myself executing these trips without a second thought, scampering along like a mountain goat and whooping at my newfound speed and sea legs.

Rowing 12+ hours every day requires a lot of fuelling, but kitchen facilities were basic at best, limited to a Jetboil (a tiny gas stove with an integrated cup), a spoon and a flask. Cooking is an elaborate description of what happened. The extent of our cooking was pouring boiling water into dehydrated meal pouches, or when we really wanted to treat ourselves, spooning peanut butter onto oatcakes. Given my job as chief water-boiler, every morning, as soon as I finished my first daylight rowing shift, I would switch to the admin area and assume my position boiling water. It was a high-stakes activity, lighting and controlling a Jetboil and then emptying the boiling contents into Stanley flasks, trying not to burn myself or anyone else. I had to keep an eye on the sea and time it right to avoid being swamped by a wave and rendering the precious Jetboil useless. Then, I'd hold the thermos and Jetboil at arm's length to transfer the water, hoping that most of it made it in. Avoiding even the smallest of injuries or skin lesions was critical, as a salty, damp environment is a breeding ground for infection and difficult to treat mid-ocean.

Toileting was a similarly hair-raising procedure, but it's extraordinary how quickly you become accustomed to performing necessary bodily functions on a precarious and highly mobile object. An ocean rowing toilet is a builder's bucket, and the process is colloquially known as "bucket and chuck it." The bucket was usually positioned in front of the third rowing position, sat opposite either Pip or Jo. An ocean rowing boat is no place for inhibitions, and having a poo became a sociable affair, sat face to face with a crew mate discussing matters of the day. Sometimes, to mix things up, usually when in a more reflective mindset or at night, we may choose a "poo with a view," facing out towards the sea, enjoying the seascape or night sky. Generally, all went well, but a sliding toilet does come with a certain degree of risk. Occasionally, a wave would catch us unawares, and we'd fly off, or worse, the chuck-it wasn't performed with sufficient care or accuracy, leaving us with a Health and Safety crisis on our hands. There were at least two incidents of "poo-gate" on board Mrs Nelson, which provided an interesting form of on-board entertainment.

Personal hygiene routines were basic but important. One of the perils to try to avoid is salt sores, which on their own can be extremely painful, but worse, can become infected and dangerous. You're frequently sprayed or drenched in salt water, so cleaning yourself as best as possible after each shift is important to minimise the risk of sores. On the whole, this is done using eco-friendly baby wipes in the privacy of the cabins, but now and again, as a treat, we'd have a bucket wash. I hasten to add that we had a second "bathroom" bucket used exclusively for washing. We'd spare a little of our precious desalinated water, slosh it into a bucket, add some multi-purpose Dr Bronner's cleaning solution, and luxuriate in the joy of a tepid rag bath. Once the bath was complete, the remaining water could be used to wash clothes. Laundry wasn't an onerous task, though, as the bulk of our daytime wardrobe (with the exception of Lebby) was pants and socks, and anything else we were happy to let fester, with the occasional salty airing on deck.

An alternative to the bucket or baby-wipe clean is nature's own shower – a rainstorm. Our weather-router, Alex Alley, an experienced Atlantic sailor, had advised us that the most practical and efficient way to wash was to wait for a storm, strip off, lather up with Dr Bronner's and let the rain wash the soap and grime away. Keen to embrace the Atlantic experience for everything it offered, I rather liked this idea and decided to give it a go.

One afternoon, I watched as the storm clouds gathered on the horizon, and the sky and sea became an ominous, saturated grey. As the first drops appeared, instead of reaching for my foulies (waterproof jacket and trousers) like the rest of the crew, I removed my clothes (it didn't take long), lathered up, and waited expectantly for the heavens to open. Unfortunately for me, the storm came to nothing more than a few pathetic drops. The Dr Bronner's lather dried on me in a sticky, white mess, much to the crew's amusement. I then had to do my best to remove the mess with a few baby wipes, and was horrified to find layer upon layer of dead skin coming off with it. My nautical exfoliation may have been efficient, but it left me surrounded by a revolting carpet of dead skin and disillusioned with the unpredictability of the weather (or my inability to predict it).

If you like your luxuries, ocean rowing is not for you. However, it's amazing how quickly you can adapt your expectations and standards of personal care and hygiene, as well as privacy and body consciousness.

Cleaning wasn't limited to ourselves or our clothes; we also had to keep Mrs Nelson ship-shape. Very occasionally, the Dr Bronners would be employed to give the deck a once-over, particularly after unfortunate bucket and chuck-it incidents, or when extreme cooking had resulted in bolognaise or korma-gate. Seeing the remnants of korma floating up and down the gunnels as the boat rose and fell with the waves was far from pleasant. Equally unpleasant were the slimy, rancid remains of flying fish, who'd tried to hitch a lift on Mrs Nelson.

An Atlantic Dip

As well as our sporadic attempts to keep the deck clean, we also had to clean the hull every week or every ten days, weather permitting. After prolonged periods in the water, barnacles and other foreign objects would grow on the hull, creating a food source for fish. The small feeding fish attract much larger, more sinister creatures, including Blue Marlin. If there's one thing you want to avoid, it's being in close proximity to one of those. They have incredibly long, sharp beaks which, on several occasions, have been known to penetrate right through the hulls of ocean rowing boats, resulting in either the boat taking on water, or the Marlin losing its beak, or both.

Cleaning the hull is a case of balancing risk and reward. On the one hand, removing barnacles reduces the risk of a Marlin strike; it makes the boat faster and allows you to stretch out your limbs in the water. On the other hand, jumping into the water and swimming around under a heavy boat, in waves, runs the risk of a blow to the head and potential injury, or worse. It's an activity which you should only attempt when conditions are conducive. Our first hull clean came on day 8 or 9, when progress was slowed by sea as still as a glassy lake. The water looked particularly inviting, so Jo and I volunteered to do the cleaning. Said cleaning involved jumping over the side into 5 km depth of water, facing who knows what sea creatures. Not to mention moving up and down the boat, diving under it with only car windscreen scrapers to remove the worst of the build-up. I hasten to add that we were tethered to the boat at all times, so we couldn't be washed away, but the adrenaline flowed, nonetheless.

I looked forward to this with a mixture of excitement and fear. I love swimming and wanted to experience the unique privilege of swimming in one of the most remote places on earth, with thousands of kilometres of ocean around me. I also have a squeamish dislike of fish, specifically fish that threaten to touch me, and a self-destructive tendency to conjure up flashbacks from particularly harrowing scenes from the 1970s film *Jaws*.

With the mantra "feel the fear and do it anyway" on repeat in my head, I gripped the woefully unstable safety line in one hand and Pip's in the other. I swung first one leg, and then the other, over the lines so that I balanced precariously on Mrs Nelson's narrow gunwale. I resisted Pip's empathetic attempts to get me to jump. I teetered and dithered on the edge, my heart pounding as I simultaneously tormented myself with images of monsters of the deep and giggled at the ludicrous predicament I had put myself in.

Realising that I was not responding to the "carrot" approach, Pip abruptly switched to the "stick" approach, and with Lebby hooting in the background and the threat of being pushed too much for my pride to take, I took an ungainly leap of faith into the unknown. As I resurfaced and adjusted my goggles, relief flooded over me. I felt the reassuring tug of my tether keeping me attached to the boat, and I allowed myself to enjoy the sensation of being in the water, my limbs revelling in the freedom of movement. But this was not a pleasure cruise; I had an important job to do.

With Pip barking instructions from the deck, I set to work with the windscreen scraper, removing the debris from the hull. After a few dives under to reach the bottom of the hull – during which I resolutely trained my eyes on the boat and *not* the inky depths below – the job was complete, and it was time to re-embark. Re-embarking is not a straightforward or elegant process. By hauling from crewmates and finding some leverage in the holes of the gunnels, we managed to slither and slide back onto deck, to the sniggers of Pip and Lebby. We'd expected to feel wonderfully clean after eight days of sweating and not showering, but instead, we looked like unkempt Smurfs. What we hadn't considered was the bright blue antifoul on Mrs Nelson's hull transferred onto anything it came into contact with, including Jo and me.

Recharging Our Batteries

Only when all necessary admin was completed could we turn our attention to the equally important job of napping. At night, it was essential to get as much sleep as possible – ideally 90 minutes each "off" shift – so that we could continue to function and maintain energy levels. During the day, napping was also important, but we each had a slightly different approach and different requirements.

It turned out that Pip and I were excellent boat-sleepers and highly skilled at falling asleep during daytime off-shifts at the drop of a hat. Daytime sleeping is something I never usually do, but I embraced it on board Mrs Nelson. I enjoyed the luxury and novelty of having a kip every few hours, lulled to sleep by the boat's gentle (or sometimes violent) rocking and the rhythmic sound of the waves slapping against the hull.

Sleep deprivation is one of the challenges of ocean rowing that we mentally prepared ourselves for. While there were some night shifts – particularly my 3 to 5 am rowing shift

– when I struggled to keep my eyes open, on the whole, I didn't feel like I suffered from a lack of sleep. I think this was partly due to my diligent approach to daytime naps, but more significantly due to our experience as mums: years of broken sleep, feeding babies through the night and knowing that you would continue to function the next day, and the next, and the next. Psychologically and physically, this gave us an advantage over crews who weren't parents, because we knew our bodies could do it, and we didn't fear sleep deprivation.

On-Board Entertainment

The monotony of eat, sleep, row, repeat may sound boring. It's one of the challenges many ocean rowers talk about and something we prepared for, but it didn't seem to trouble The Mothership. The prospect of being bored is something I relished because it would mean we had time to think and breathe, time that wasn't immediately consumed by the next job on the list or the loudest voice in the room.

We'd all taken Kindles with us, imagining we'd have time on our hands to read and would want some form of entertainment to stave off the boredom. But they were quickly relegated to the farthest corners of the hatches – one of the items cited in one of our final social media posts as the "most useless piece of kit on an ocean rowing boat."

The truth was that we embraced the time we had just to *be*, savouring the opportunity to let our minds wander, think, daydream and be quietly entertained by the subtle but ever-changing world around us.

It's amazing how you rekindle your imagination when you're released from all the distractions of modern life, particularly technology and screens. Creativity flows, and you find endless activities to fill the void.

I lost hours just watching the changing patterns of the waves, mesmerised by the endless, repeating motion – the rise and fall of the water and the way the light revealed a thousand different colours in it as night turned to day and day turned to night. During daylight, the sky was another avenue of entertainment. Over the course of a shift, we'd give a running commentary on how the clouds morphed into different objects, from polar bears and ducks to Formula 1 cars and countries. We'd watch the clouds form and multiply on the horizon, wondering whether that signalled a storm or the ever-elusive and longed-for trade winds.

It wasn't just imaginary cloud-animals that provided entertainment. Some of our most magical moments during those 40 days were our encounters with the other lives around us.

If there was an element of the row that didn't live up to expectation, it was the sea life. I think we'd all imagined that the Atlantic would be teeming with life. If not a constant source of entertainment, then at least a regular flow of interest in the form of dolphins, whales, turtles, fish, perhaps even sharks. I'd rather whimsically imagine whale tails in the distance, the sound of water and air erupting from blowholes and families of turtles bobbing in the waves. And in the dead of night in the early days of training, my mind would conjure up images from *Jaws*, with the gruesome, angular jaws of a great white rearing out of the water, ready to swallow our boat whole. I knew the drill: stuff a fire extinguisher into its mouth, and all would be well.

In reality, however, days and days would pass with nothing much to see in the vast ocean around us. In retrospect, I suspect there was a lot more to see if we'd known how to look for it. The scarcity of sightings probably made those moments all the more thrilling, and the fin of a dolphin would cause a ripple of shrieks from the boat, heads frantically gesturing in the relevant direction. (With both hands on the oars, head movements were a reliable substitute for pointing.)

On one occasion, we were surrounded by dolphins, hundreds of beautiful, graceful creatures swimming alongside, underneath, and all around us, appearing to leap and dive for the sheer joy of it. It was almost as if they'd spotted us from afar and come to welcome us to their playground, accompanying us for a short but very sweet portion of our journey. Those were moments we treasured, moments that lifted our spirits, lightened our souls and left us glowing with the memory of our privileged glimpse into the beauty of a world so few people ever experience.

Crew Conversation: From Politics to Profanities

If nature provided spikes of excitement and motivation, conversation was the fuel that kept us pushing along. We thought we'd ticked off "get to know your crewmates" through training, but it's when you have hours, and hours, and hours and hours to talk that you realise you've only been scratching the surface. Sometimes we'd share more intimate conversations with our rowing buddy, at other times we'd enjoy full-crew debates. The beauty of having a split shift pattern, with a change of rower every hour, was that there was always a fresh conversation to begin, or a different perspective on the existing debate.

One of the things I treasure most about the whole experience of the row was the time I spent with Pip. You'd have thought we knew each other inside and out, having grown up together and remained close in adulthood. Looking back, though, I'm not sure we ever spent that much time in such close proximity, with endless time to talk about all elements of life. And it was a joy – one of the greatest privileges of the row. Pip is a mum of four, and life is usually hectic, juggling far too many balls. To see Pip in a completely different environment, with life stripped back to the basics and free of all the stressors of normal life, was wonderful. For all of us, it was like peeling back the layers of life and reconnecting with the people we really are, deep down, before life adds its inevitable influence.

Conversation flowed freely, and we explored countless topics, from high-brow, broadsheet-worthy intellectual discussion to frivolous, raucous tales that not even the gutter press would print. Jo and Lebby are brilliant raconteurs, and entire shifts could go by with Pip and I regaled by hilarious stories from their past, leaving us doubled over, not from the effort of rowing, but from the effort of laughing. To offer a piece of advice to anyone considering rowing an ocean or undertaking any other lengthy challenge, choose your companions wisely. Those with a past, ideally a colourful past, will be a tremendous entertainment asset.

And when we weren't sharing intimate stories or coming up with answers to world peace, we'd revert to good, old-fashioned entertainment in the form of word games. We played countless rounds of the ABC game, ranging from family favourites like sandwich fillings and film titles, to the "after the watershed" options, including profanities and past "conquests." It's incredible how obscene you can be when under pressure to find an "s", and the names of old flames you can dredge from your memory vaults when required. I will forever be impressed and amazed in equal measure by one crew member's ability to run through the entire alphabet of conquests on her own. (Yes, even "Q" and "X".)

Night-Life

Boat life took on a different mantle at night, and the experience hinged on the weather conditions. For the first few nights, the moon eased our passage through the ocean. I had never consciously observed moonrises before, but they were stunning. These first few nights had lulled us into a false sense of security about what nighttime would be like.

With the moon out, our passage was bathed in bright light, almost like a pathway lit to guide us. It was serene and beautiful, especially with a sky overflowing with twinkling stars, shooting stars and satellites. We could see clearly with the deck illuminated by the moon, and life was relatively easy.

After a few nights, we started to notice that the moon was becoming a little tardy, displaying a disappointing work ethic. It was inconvenient, to say the least, because rowing in the pitch black is a very different kettle of fish. You can no longer see what's around you, you can't anticipate the arrival of waves or brace yourself for the soaking. And after a while, the moon stopped showing up for work altogether, leaving us rowing in the inky darkness all night.

We were disappointed, outraged and perplexed. For four intelligent and capable women, this adventure had exposed a gaping hole in our knowledge: a complete and utter ignorance of the moon's movement and astronomy in general.

After several shifts discussing this peculiar phenomenon, I swallowed my pride and emailed Paul to ask for enlightenment. I felt marginally better when I found out he didn't know either and had to send us Google's explanation. Although I still can't explain why, I now know that the moon rises and sets at different times of the night and day, so sometimes it doesn't appear at all during the nighttime.

When the moon was taking a sickie and the waves were big, rowing at night was like riding a magic carpet or hurtling, out of control, through a black-hole rollercoaster. We had no idea which way we would lurch at any point – up, down, right or left. Countless shifts blurred into the same hair-raising experience, my hands gripping the oars tightly, knuckles stretched white, jaw clenched, ears and eyes straining, desperately trying to anticipate where the next wave was coming from.

We'd carry on rowing because it was the only thing to do, but sometimes our oars would miss the water entirely and thrash wildly in the air, or clash with the rower in front, causing a disgruntled glance backwards. Sometimes the oars would come crashing down on our shins, resulting in yelps of pain and cursing, carried away on the wind. During those shifts, I'd wait anxiously for shift change, then clamber back into the relative sanctity of the cabin and feel the tension finally release from my body, to be replaced by all-encompassing exhaustion.

Night-time rowing was bliss at other times, with clear moonlit skies and more gentle waves. It was a time for quieter contemplation, and there were moments when I'd look to the heavens and feel overwhelmed by the beauty and power of the world around us – the endless magnificence of the sky, the luminous reflection of the moon on the sea, the coolness of the sea breeze refreshing our skin. I felt an all-encompassing gratitude for being there and having the opportunity to experience something so extraordinary. I loved those nights.

Sometimes we'd chat, sometimes we'd get lost in our thoughts and sometimes we'd listen to music and sing at the tops of our voices. Occasionally, we'd struggle to stay awake, and then it was the responsibility of the least exhausted to keep conversation flowing or intermittently prod the other to wake up. When you were sitting in the bow seat, it was easy to spot when your rowing partner had lost the battle with sleep. But if you were in the front, it was the sudden silence or the repeated clashing of oars that alerted you to a slumbering teammate.

Above all else, 40 days in our little ocean rowing boat, with life pared back to the bare minimum, taught me how to find joy in just *being*. It taught me to flourish in an alien but simple environment and to appreciate the world and the people around me.

In modern life, we surround ourselves with things we think we need to make our lives better – possessions, clutter, activities, technology, entertainment. Only when these things are stripped away do you appreciate how little you need in life to feel fulfilled and deeply content.

Chapter 8
Rowing Through Storms

The race is now called "The World's Toughest Row" for good reason. While some of what I've described may make it sound like a pleasure cruise, that reflects my approach and mindset toward the experience more than the experience itself. From day one, it was far from plain sailing.

"Expect the unexpected" is a great motto to take with you into any challenge. An Atlantic row is no different. We'd trained for endless scenarios but knew we'd also have to face things we hadn't trained for, things that would call on our initiative, reserves and ability to respond in a high-pressure situation. We trained to tackle the unexpected.

In some ways, the weather was kind to us in our first few days, with reasonably light winds, dawn-to-dusk sunshine and calm seas. The weather meant sea sickness was mild (Pip may beg to differ on this point), and we could acclimatise to our new environment relatively easily, without the peril of a pitching boat or the inconvenience and discomfort of being permanently wet. As experienced river rowers, the calm seas played to our natural inclination to keep a good rowing technique – staying in time, keeping our balance, taking full strokes and holding our finishes. But there is a flip side to every coin.

Calm seas, as we were to find out, are sticky seas. With little advantage from wind or waves, and a heavy boat laden with 55 days of supplies, it was like we were rowing through treacle. Rowing was as demanding as weightlifting, each stroke taking its toll on our bodies. Progress was slow, and picking up a satisfactory pace was impossible. The slow progress quickly boiled over into frustration. We were experienced rowers, and we couldn't understand why we couldn't make the boat go faster. Surely we must be doing something wrong?

We'd have endless discussions about what we could do differently. Should we shift some weight? Was our tech on the wrong setting? Should we have the centreboard up or down? We became obsessed with the boat's speed, watching the deck repeater and willing the numbers to tick up, doing mental boat maths to work out how long it might take us at the current rate. The answer was never a good one, and it tested all our collective optimism and belief. We all started to wonder whether we had bitten off more than we could chew, and whether our lofty aspiration to complete the race in under 45 days was simply the pie-in-the-sky dreaming of delusional wannabes. It certainly knocked some of the wind out of our sails.

Despite our concerted efforts, nothing we did made any difference to our speed, and we had to come to terms with the fact that we were just going more slowly than we'd hoped, and it might take a little longer to get to Antigua than we'd planned. We had to find a way of controlling the frustration and putting our faith in our processes so that even though we might be going more slowly, we were a little closer to our goal with each stroke. If we put our heads down and carried on chipping away, we would get there. We had to forget about the finish line and the boat maths and concentrate on doing the best we could in the moment, given the conditions we had. It was the best thing we could do.

The combination of heavy seas and our bodies getting used to the relentless strain of rowing for 12+ hours every day soon led to some physical niggles. Our hands were the first to show signs of friction and wear. Blisters erupted and burst, and our skin turned red, hot and tender before they toughened and grew immune to the daily grind. Necks, shoulders and backs took turns begging for mercy, and with each shift change, we'd have a new ailment to ponder.

I started to lose my vision, or more specifically, my ability to focus on detail. This is a common side effect of sea sickness patches, but it was the lesser of two evils, so I persevered until the threat of sea sickness had abated. It was an odd but minor inconvenience, as I'd quickly realised that we wouldn't be devouring novels, and I knew it was temporary.

Unexpected Encounters

During our second night on board, as we were getting used to our routines and finding our feet, our first major challenge presented itself. My alarm broke through my sleep – my signal to force myself up to sitting, pull on socks, pants and a top, and crawl out onto deck for my shift. Although early in the row, we'd got used to peace and calm on deck at night. Opening the cabin door, I was confronted with a different scene. Ordinarily, I would have swapped with Lebby and joined Jo on the oars while Pip slept, but instead I found all three on deck in animated conversation, gesticulating towards the lights of a nearby boat. (As a side note, having any other vessel nearby in the Atlantic is unusual.)

While I'd been peacefully sleeping, the rest of the crew had been dealing with an emergency. Pip's sleep had been interrupted by the Automatic Identification System (AIS) alarm sounding, indicating another boat was in close proximity to us and on a collision course. Pip had tried to radio the boat with no response, and with the much larger, faster vessel heading straight for us, had set off a white flare, hoping to arouse their attention. Fortunately, it did the trick, and as I clambered out onto deck, the lights were heading away from us, the boat having course-corrected. Disaster averted, Pip and Lebby retreated into the cabins and normal service resumed.

While the air of excitement and adrenaline continued through my shift, as first Jo and then Pip debriefed me on the incident, the tale was also recounted with an element of pride. We'd passed our first big test: how to react in an emergency, follow protocol and keep ourselves safe. We'd practised our radio drill and flare drill, grateful for our training, and as a result of coming through it all safely, we were visibly more confident in our ability to handle challenges.

Four hours later, rubbing the sleep from my eyes as I cracked open the cabin door for my next shift, I could have been forgiven for thinking time had got stuck in an unfortunate loop. The deck was alive with agitated activity, and everyone else was already there – Jo and Lebby were going through the motions of rowing. At the same time, Pip stood, radio in hand, looking over the stern towards the lights of an even larger approaching vessel. Surely this couldn't be happening again!

There's nothing like a bit of drama to shake off the shadows of sleep, and I was soon wide awake, all senses alert. But this was a different challenge. Although a boat was clearly heading directly towards us, it was not showing on our AIS, which meant we couldn't identify or radio it. It didn't take long for the reality of this latest predicament to sink in. If we didn't get its attention, we'd be fish fodder – and not wishing to run through our entire supply of white flares in one night, we decided to phone a friend for some advice.

The race safety team is available 24/7 for advice or a friendly ear when needed. And we needed it. After a quick conversation with Safety HQ, Pip put out an anonymous call on the radio, audible to any boat within range, as Jo, Lebby and I watched and waited, hearts in mouths. After a few moments of agonising silence, the radio crackled to life and a Spanish voice answered. Switching to a closed channel, Pip quickly explained who we were and where we were, and politely but insistently asked him to change course.

The captain of the approaching Spanish naval ship was extremely obliging and jolly. In an amused tone and thickly accented English, he reassured Pip that he could see us and told her, "It doesn't matter." It did matter – to us, *a lot* – and for the second time in one night, it was with a collective sigh of relief that we watched the lights slowly turn and the dark hulk of the huge ship slip away into the darkness. Disaster averted, again.

These may sound like alarming incidents, and the consequences of not effectively managing them could have been catastrophic. But if it was a test of how to handle pressure, we all passed with flying colours. Even with the AIS alarm becoming increasingly persistent and agitated, we kept our heads. We focused not on catastrophising, but on the steps we needed to take to eliminate danger, including asking for help.

Pride can sometimes prevent us from asking for help, but it's a critical tool in our survival toolbox. An ocean rowing boat is no place for pride and ego, and knowing when – and who – to ask for help was one of our greatest strengths.

Our ability to stay calm under pressure and work together as a team is a testament to the rigorous training over the previous two years. Incidents like these are why we go through mandatory training courses, practise drills during training, run through different scenarios, spend time learning how each other operates and are tested on our knowledge and equipment before we're declared safe to race. Our training and preparation have given us the skills and attitude to tackle unforeseen challenges and emerge stronger.

Having anticipated not coming into close contact – or possibly even laying eyes on – another boat for the duration of our crossing, two close encounters in one night were far from expected. It tested our mettle, nerves, ability to react under pressure, teamwork, resourcefulness and training.

While we each handled the pressure slightly differently, what made me most proud was how we handled it as a team. It brought us together, not apart, each of us playing our role to get us through. Lebby and I took the oars so that Pip and

Jo could lead on steering and communications. We supported each other. Jo's calmness and ability to keep a clear head, combined with Pip's humour, were a welcome tonic to the pressure of the situation. Lebby and I could channel the pressure through the oars.

Of course, we were relieved to have navigated the challenges safely, but the sense of pride it gave us – and the novelty of having had such excitement in what is usually such a monotonous routine – visibly lifted us all, a tangible energy flowing through the crew.

We'd passed our first significant test. We felt a little more like gnarly ocean rowers; we'd grown in confidence and were ready to face whatever challenges lay ahead.

Compete or Complete?

The next challenge was as unexpected as it was significant and permeated a large portion of our crossing and our approach to it. The World's Toughest Row is a race, but like many extreme endurance events, not everyone is in it to win it. For the majority, achievement and satisfaction lie in the experience of taking part and completing the race, rather than being pegged on a time or position. For most crews, it becomes a question of "compete or complete." In our case, we fell somewhere in the middle. We aimed to complete the race as fast as we could, to the best of our ability, in a way we could be proud of, while making the most of this unique experience. We weren't interested in competing against other crews for the win at the expense of the experience and crew dynamics.

Our crew motto was "Stay safe, stay friends, stay strong." Safety was paramount because we were responsible to each other and to our families to minimise risk and return home safely. Staying friends was critical: the extremes of ocean rowing often expose and create divides within crews, breaking down relationships and making the journey something to endure rather than enjoy. We knew how much everyone around us had sacrificed to enable us to do this, and we were determined to make the most of the experience and return as lifelong friends. Staying strong was about doing everything we could to be mentally and physically robust to support each other and achieve our potential, but it wasn't about speed at all costs. That would have meant approaching the race differently, and for us, it would have felt detrimental to the experience and our team values.

We hadn't even researched our "competitors" in the race because it wasn't something that was important to us or that we thought would affect our preparation or approach. However, being thrown into a different environment can bring out buried traits, and the Atlantic unleashed our competitive instinct.

Each rowing boat is fitted with a tracking device, which enables the race organisers, as well as anyone else interested, to monitor progress across the ocean, with four-hourly updates. Each boat is represented by a dot on the tracking app, and "dot watching" becomes an endurance event in its own right. While those at home can monitor each boat's position at the touch of a button, we could only monitor our position on the boats through updates from land support. It's difficult to get a clear picture of race positions in the first few days, as each boat takes a different route, but after a while, when everyone has settled into their routines, the leaderboard begins to take shape.

Despite our slow progress in the early days, we were delighted to hear we were making excellent headway in the fleet and were neck and neck for the lead in the women's race with another female four, One Ocean Crew, albeit hundreds of miles apart, having chosen different bearings leaving La Gomera. This news boosted our confidence and fuelled the competitive spirit in each of us – a spirit kindled by One Ocean Crew a couple of days before the race began. In their pre-race interview, they spoke about their aim to win the women's race, and the result was like poking a bear. We were indignant and quietly amused by being disregarded by our much more youthful competitors, and we filed that away in our motivation bank, determined to give them a run for their money.

Finding out we were in a competitive position was a turning point in our race, because suddenly it wasn't just about us and what we were doing – it was about One Ocean Crew, and what we imagined they might be doing. And that was entirely out of our control. Occasional calls home became daily or twice-daily occurrences for Lebby, whose children still maintain that the only reason she ever called home was to find out our latest position. Lebby would poke her head out of the cabin to broadcast the outcome of those calls, which would inevitably affect the mood onboard. Disappointment when we'd lost a mile or two boiled over into frustration. We were slogging our guts out, confident in our strength, but why couldn't we push ahead?

This new and unexpected dynamic also revealed differences between our individual approaches to the race and our competitive nature. Although we'd agreed that we wouldn't race at all costs, this new drive meant we had to review that. To a greater or lesser degree, we all wanted to show everyone what four middle-aged mums in a boat were capable of, and we wanted to prove the naysayers wrong, including our younger rivals. But were we prepared to change our approach to make a point?

We reviewed our options: carry on as we were, row our race as planned or change tactics to try to compete for the women's race win. We couldn't ignore our gut reaction or the daily updates' effect on morale. For the greater good of the team dynamics and staying true to our mantra to "stay safe, stay friends, stay strong," we collectively agreed to adapt our approach and try to row faster.

This change had a significant impact on our routines. Rowing faster meant rowing "3-up" – three people rowing together instead of two – during daylight hours, reducing our daylight rest shifts to just one hour. It was brutal, but just about sustainable. Crucially, it was an element we could control. Our boat speed increased, and with it, we started to gain ground on One Ocean Crew. The ongoing battle for the lead continued and became a prominent feature of our experience. It added an unexpected – but not unwelcome – dimension to our race, giving us a new focus outside the usual routine, a new topic of conversation, a more immediate target, and a motivation to dig deeper each shift and drive ourselves forward. We settled into our new routine, embracing the dynamic, relishing the thrill of the chase, and becoming accustomed to the highs and lows of the morning and evening position updates.

Eventually, after plugging away in our new routine for a few days, we were rewarded around New Year when our morning update showed we'd taken a healthy lead. Suddenly, it felt like we were pulling away, and we were jubilant. But pride comes before a fall, and races like this aren't won overnight. One Ocean Crew responded and began chipping away at our lead – chipping away at our confidence, too – eventually regaining the lead. As they nudged ahead, mile by painful mile, with a few hundred miles and a few days left to go, we knew we had to change tactics again if we were going to win. We couldn't understand how they could go faster when we were giving it everything. We tried to find reasons, other than crew strength and resilience, to explain the difference: boat weight, kit, weather. But in the end, this only served to torment us, and we'll never know what difference, if any, those things made. The only thing left that we could influence was how much we rowed, and the only way we could see to gain an advantage was to row more, row 3-up at night and during the day.

We discussed this as a crew and agreed to give it a go. It would mean each of us rowing for 18 hours every 24 hours, getting four to five hours of sleep if we were lucky.

It was not a fruitful experiment. It was neither sustainable nor productive. We didn't gain any ground during that first night, and to make matters worse, we felt the effects the following day. Lebby had particularly struggled, hallucinating and regularly falling asleep on the oars. We realised it was counterproductive to performance, wellbeing and crew dynamics to continue like that.

But we had nothing left to give, no aces left to play. Reluctantly, we had to concede that, in all likelihood, this wasn't a race we would win. Although disappointing to have been so close for so long, liberating ourselves from the pressure of the race and the twice-daily updates was a relief in many ways. It gave us the opportunity to refocus our efforts on a goal that didn't depend on the efforts of another team.

We picked ourselves up and set a new target: reaching Antigua for sundown drinks on Friday, January 21, 40 days after setting out from La Gomera. It still meant pushing on and challenging ourselves, but it was back to being about the four of us in the boat, as it had been at the start.

With The Mothership and One Ocean Crew racing neck and neck for thousands of miles over several weeks, it was hard to admit we were beaten, particularly for Lebby, whose competitive edge ran deepest. However, we could take pride in how we'd worked together, adapted, dug deep and pushed ourselves further than we could ever have imagined. Eventually, we arrived in Antigua just a few hours after One Ocean Crew, but it still felt like a victory.

We donned our caps to One Ocean Crew because the grit, determination and resilience we'd shown over thousands of miles had been matched, and more, by those plucky four women. We knew what it must have taken to win the race, and we celebrated that. It was a victory for One Ocean Crew and a victory for women.

Winning the race had never been our dream or goal, but it was an opportunity that presented itself along the way, and something we seized. Sometimes life doesn't go according to plan. Different routes emerge, and we have choices to make. Progress isn't about rigidly sticking to plans, but about adapting and flexing according to the situation you're faced with. And that's what we did.

Stormy Seas

As the race-within-a-race with One Ocean Crew picked up pace, so did the weather, and we moved from the nursery slopes of the Atlantic into terrifying black runs. Conditions can change with the flip of a coin at sea, and one day, a couple of weeks into the race, I climbed out of my cabin and, looking around, felt like I'd emerged into a different world. The glassy sea had transformed into a swirling cauldron of grey, with what looked like huge but choppy waves making the boat pitch and roll. I needed to get to the other end of the boat to use the bucket and wondered how I would navigate this hairy journey. It probably wasn't pretty or gainly, but I made it, proud of my efforts.

The new views were alarming at first, and the new movement of the boat took a little getting used to, but it wasn't long before I found myself enjoying the thrill. This was what we'd signed up for. I'd been terrified of the prospect of the big waves when I first agreed to the race, but now I was in the middle of them and enjoying it. It was a refreshing contrast to the pace and slog of the first few days, and as we felt the boat moving faster, we willed the wind to pick up further and the waves to carry us higher.

We experimented with surfing the waves, learning at what point to stop rowing and let the momentum of the boat and the wave carry us down into the valleys, before rowing again to pull us up the next crest. I'm not sure we ever mastered it, but it was fun trying.

The downside of the big seas was the battering our shins took. The pain of it was something nobody had warned us about, but it was excruciating and absolutely unavoidable. The most exasperating thing was that you could see it coming, knew you were about to fall victim to a beating, but could do absolutely nothing to stop it. During high seas, there would be intermittent cries from one or another rower, as yet again an oar slammed down on their shins. Sometimes we mustered the energy to curse and shout; sometimes it was more of a pathetic whimper as we accepted our fate.

We developed a new vernacular for the shin-slamming action, correlating with particular types of waves and the corresponding motion of the oars. From the slam-dunk to the karate chop, they were all malicious, but the worst was probably the "pass the baton," which had a double-whammy effect of first impacting the shin, before being dragged backwards, scraping the hip bone. The motion would leave the unfortunate rower with one arm contorted behind their back, appearing to pass the baton to the rower behind. Pip was in so much pain one day that she resorted to fashioning a pair of shin pads from a leftover yoga mat. She looked ridiculous, but when you're closer to astronauts on the International Space Station than to other people on land, what you look like is the last thing you need to worry about.

The rest of us were hardly in a position to preach about fashion choices. I'd opted for the minimalist look from hour two of day one, with trainers, socks, pants and a visor being my outfit of choice for most shifts. Jo favoured a similar look, with the addition of a vest that could stand up on its own after weeks of not being washed. Lebby was the outlier, choosing the protective approach, with leggings, a long-sleeved shirt and a floppy hat covering every inch of skin. At night, even in 20-plus degrees, she would swap the hat for a beanie. When we arrived in Antigua with remarkably contrasting skin tones, one of the questions that popped up on our Instagram feed was whether Lebby had only rowed night shifts.

As we adapted to a more turbulent ocean and saw how Mrs Nelson could handle big waves, rising and falling effortlessly with each crest, leaning and tipping as if in sync with, rather than battling, the water, we gained confidence and began to make more rapid progress. With that, our confidence grew: confidence in our ability to handle whatever the Atlantic might offer and Mrs Nelson's ability to handle it, too.

Sometimes our biggest fears are in our heads. The fear of the unknown can be overwhelming; it can stop us from doing things. Only when we push and challenge ourselves to face those fears does the unknown become familiar, the fear disappears, and we realise how capable we are. Facing my fear of the waves wasn't just a case of leaping into a boat and heading out into the ocean. It was the product of nearly two years of training, mentally adjusting to the notion of what might lie ahead, visualising being in the thick of giant waves, learning about the boat's design and ability to navigate safely, accepting waves as a reality and not something that would hold us back but instead push us forward more quickly to our goal.

Those first days of choppy seas were just the appetiser in the Atlantic's menu of treats. Alongside waves, we had to learn to adapt to storms and squalls, including the heaviest rain I have ever experienced.

We'd had three weeks of staying mostly dry, with no need to dig out our foulies for protection. Suddenly, our foulies were in and out of their dry bags regularly, as the changing weather brought short, sharp showers as well as livid storms.

Jo and I were on shift one day when the first major squall hit us. We'd seen the clouds forming, the sky becoming an ominous, deep, heavy grey, and an eerie stillness fell. It was the lull before the storm. The heavens opened, and the rain lashed down so hard it hurt any exposed skin, bouncing off everything it touched. We hunched over our oars, eyes squinting both to try to see through the rain and protect our eyes from the needle-like onslaught. The noise was overwhelming, and we had to shout to have any hope of hearing each other. With the rain came fierce wind, sending us careening through the daytime darkness faster than ever. We were completely at the will of the wind and sea. Battling it would have been futile, so we just had to row with it and hope we wouldn't be pushed too far off course when it passed.

The adrenaline was pumping hard, and for the first time, we were experiencing the fear of being at the mercy of the mighty Atlantic. Jo yelled over her shoulder to me, "Just hold on and keep rowing!"

"I am!" I retorted. I gripped the oars as tightly as I could, knuckles white, holding on for dear life and wondering how long this would last.

As it continued, and again we realised what we and Mrs Nelson could cope with, the fear turned to laughter. We were laughing at our tiny insignificance against the will of Mother Nature, laughing at the ridiculous situation we'd chosen to put ourselves in, laughing in awe of our capacity to cope and our spirit in adversity, and laughing with relief that it didn't seem like we'd be propelled out of the boat into the swirling water.

The squall ran out of energy as quickly as it had built, and when the rain abated to a few gentle drops, I heard the cabin door behind me creak open, and Lebby poked her head out. "Are you OK?" she asked cautiously. Happily, we were all smiling, pumped by the experience.

As I later learned, being inside a cabin during a squall is no picnic either. If it's loud on deck, it's louder in the cabin. As the rain pelts down on the roof, the waves pummel the sides and the wind howls across the boat. The cabin door is taped up with reflective bubble wrap to keep the sun out, so you can't see outside, and you can't risk opening the door to find out what's happening. Your imagination starts running wild, fearing the worst. Sleep is pretty futile during these conditions, so you have to wait it out, taking small comfort in the fact that you're warm and dry while your rowing buddies are cold to the bone and drenched – either from the skies, the sea, or most likely, both.

With each new challenge or obstacle we encountered, we learned more about our individual, as well as our collective, responses to pressure and the implications of our reactions for the different roles we played in high-pressure situations. Our positions in the boat also naturally determined how we slotted in.

Pip and Jo were based in the stern cabin, which was also the hub for most of our technical equipment and data, including navigation, steering and batteries. Lebby and I dossed down in the bow cabin, palatial by comparison, but lacking in "kit" and so could feel isolating. Owing to its superior size, the bow cabin soon became a dumping ground for equipment we couldn't squeeze elsewhere and debris from half-eaten meals, snacks and sweaty underwear. Even a teenage boy's room couldn't have competed on smell, and the affectionate name "The Hovel" was coined.

Although the boat is small, traversing up and down can be hazardous and disruptive, so we limited it to the minimum. As a result, Lebby and I were relative strangers to the screens, bleeps and flashes of the stern cabin and far less equipped to deal with technical issues. When problems arose, we typically defaulted to the boat's brawn, hauling away at the oars and taking instruction from the brains – Pip and Jo.

Jo was cool as a cucumber under pressure, able to stay calm and focus on logically working through a problem. When you need to get yourself out of a tight fix, there's no one I'd rather have on my side. We'd seen this during training, when she took the lead during our ill-advised game of chicken with passenger ferries in Portsmouth Harbour, and she came into her own when the Atlantic threw its toys.

Pip epitomised versatility. As skipper, she was comfortable leading from the front and working alongside Jo to figure out a problem, but equally happy to slot into position on the oars and add to the brawn, if that's how she could contribute more.

Lebby was the powerhouse and would naturally channel any pressure she felt into power through the oars. Deeply competitive, the Atlantic posed an excellent sparring partner and often bore the brunt of her spirit.

I was the steadier and smaller half of the brawn – calm under pressure, stubbornly optimistic, head down and resolutely plugging away until the job was done, finding comfort in having a purpose on the oars.

High-pressure environments call for calm, decisive action and putting individual egos aside. There's time afterwards for lengthy debate and analysis, but in the heat of the moment, someone needs to step up and lead, and others need to rally around and work together as a unit to complete the task. As my mum often said – and I've learned from my experience of overseeing three budding chefs – you can't have too many cooks in the kitchen.

Chapter 9
The Nightmare Before Christmas

Heavy seas, close encounters with ghost ships, the psychological strain of the race with One Ocean Crew and Atlantic squalls were the warm-up acts for the main event. They were the Atlantic's way of getting us to flex our mental and physical muscles so that we were ready and prepared for when it unleashed its full might and power.

Christmas was always going to be a tough time on board. As it's usually a time spent with family, as mums, it's when we felt the absence of our children most acutely. Christmas on the boat was a very different experience: no creeping into bedrooms to lay out the stockings; no children jumping on the bed far too early to announce that Father Christmas had been; no wide-eyed wonder at the pile of presents under the tree; no table groaning with food; no fizz before lunch; no Quality Street; no posh frocks or Christmas jumpers.

Nevertheless, we were determined to enjoy Christmas in our own way and to mark it as a day different from the others on board.

However, life rarely goes according to plan, particularly not life on a small boat mid-Atlantic. Things started unravelling at lunchtime on Christmas Eve. As was customary, at around midday, halfway through my shift, I took a quick break to arrange the water canisters so we could turn on the water maker and replenish our clean water supply. Lebby was on standby in the cabin behind me, ready to power on the water maker. At the same time, I listened out for the characteristic "clunk" and made sure that everything was functioning as it should, with clean water filling the canisters while wastewater poured into the gunnels.

"Okay!" shouted Lebby to indicate that the power was on, but there was no reassuring clunk from the water maker, and neither clean water nor wastewater came out. Although it's not unusual for water makers to malfunction, it's still one of the scenarios you dread, because life at sea without a functioning automatic water maker is very challenging, sometimes row-ending.

Lebby and I, collectively responsible for all things water, turned our attention to trying to fix it. There is a standard operating procedure to follow when your water maker stops working. Usually, it's because air has been sucked into the mechanism, and there's a simple process for clearing the airlock. However, in this case, after consulting our laminated guide and methodically working through the steps, the reassuring clunk still eluded us.

As the smallest person on the boat, I was designated "hatch mouse" and ferreted around half in, half out of the water maker hatch, trying to work out the problem. It's not a pleasant place to be. With temperatures on deck in the high 30s, it's even hotter in the depths of the hatches. Upside down, with blood running to my head, I struggled to see through the sweat stinging my eyes.

After some basic initial investigation, we deduced that since there was no water coming out, there was probably also no water coming in – so perhaps there was a blockage in the inlet pipe. Having tried and failed to remove it with some fairly forceful tugging, and not wanting to risk terminally damaging the precious machine, we decided it was time for backup and phoned the race safety team.

Agreeing with our diagnosis, they advised us to be more forceful in removing the inlet pipe. After much more sweating, swearing, and tugging – head down in the smelly, damp hatch – we finally managed to remove the pipe, ensure it was free from blockage, and reattach it.

After a couple of very nervous, tense hours of amateur diagnostics and mechanics, it was time for the moment of truth. Once again, I gave Lebby the nod. She powered up the machine, and after a few seconds, which felt more like minutes, our water maker once more spluttered into life with a resounding clunk, followed shortly by the beautiful sight of water flowing into the canister and out of the waste pipe.

It was with a mixture of not inconsiderable pride and relief that I resumed my position on the oars, relieving Jo from her double shift. Lebby retreated into The Hovel for a snack, and we settled back into our routines, for a while at least.

My attention turned to the pressing matter of Christmas, and how to mark this unique experience of Christmas bobbing around on a tiny little boat. One of my favourite Christmas traditions, influenced by my Mum, is *Carols from King's* on Christmas Eve – hearing the moving sound of the soloist choirboy singing "Once in Royal David's City" against the backdrop of the usual Christmas Eve chaos of a busy family household. It's the only time I ever remember Mum taking a break from preparations, and she'd try desperately to hear it over the din of everything else that was going on.

Along with the carols were the nine lessons telling the Christmas story – something so familiar yet incredibly difficult to piece together when you actually want to. Pip and I discussed the content at length, failing miserably to cobble together a coherent tale beyond the basic story, despite over 40 years of hearing it.

Undeterred, we decided to celebrate Christmas with a makeshift Midnight Mass, which would start when I came on shift at 11 p.m. and continue for as long as we had the energy or words for carols – at least long enough to welcome in Christmas Day. There's nothing like a good sing-along at the tops of your lungs to lift the spirits, entertaining no one other than yourselves and any nature in earshot.

I was quite sure that Mum and Dad would heartily approve of the intent – if not our interpretation of the nine lessons – and I was very much looking forward to donning my Santa hat and beginning my 11 pm shift.

Alas, things didn't work out quite as I'd hoped.

My alarm sounded and I sat up, with rather more vim and vigour than usual, and pulled on my night uniform of pants, socks and long-sleeved top. The Santa hat evaded my half-hearted search in the dimly lit cabin, but figuring I'd get too hot anyway, I nudged open the cabin door to let Lebs know I was ready for changeover.

However, rather than the usual muted conversation, the deck was a hive of activity and raised voices, with Pip, who should have been sleeping, on the oars with Lebby. Jo was intermittently popping out of the stern cabin like a jack-in-the-box to check the latest conditions and assess the situation.

As I emerged, I pieced together strands of conversation including "fish," "rudder," "steering," "waves," "we have to turn the boat," and quickly concluded that all was not well. Facial expressions said it all: furrowed brows, the grimace of physical exertion, flashing eyes anxiously scanning the blackness, faces turned expectantly towards Jo every time she emerged, hoping for an answer and some respite. *Silent Night* it was not. It was no time for my nine lessons and carols. Christmas cheer was not in abundance.

During my slumber, the wind had picked up pace, whipping the sea into a frenzy. (It must have wreaked havoc with Santa's sleigh ride.) As well as now having to contend with unpredictable waves, we were also battling with a shoal of flying fish, who seemed keen on hitching a lift on the boat rather than taking their chances with the waves.

Amidst all this, something had impacted our steering, which appeared to have locked in the wrong position. We were spinning out of control – the boat was turning the wrong way in the water, with the waves attacking us side-on. This situation is not something you ever want to find yourself in, as it's the most unstable position for the boat, and there's a reasonable chance of capsizing.

In the confusion, working out what had gone wrong was impossible. Theories ranged from a huge shoal of flying fish somehow jamming the rudder to a large wave, an unknown object, a sea creature snapping the rudder or the autohelm locking in the wrong position.

Regardless of the cause, the immediate priority was safety and trying to turn the boat back around – far easier said than done when pitted against Atlantic waves and wind. I slotted into my usual seat in the bow, while Lebby moved to the stern so we could row 3-up. We battled away for a couple of hours, and most of the time, it was like putting our oars into concrete, with barely any leverage in the water. Jo monitored the tech and continued to work on the cause, shouting encouragement as required, until eventually, Mrs Nelson was facing the right way again, the stars were back where they should be in the sky, and we began to make more stable progress in the intended direction.

For all of us, it was probably the most alarming time of the crossing. We faced the danger of capsizing with the boat pointing in the wrong direction. But worse than that for me was the fear of the unknown mechanical problem and its potential consequences. In the dead of night, with the wind and waves howling and crashing, we couldn't work out what had gone wrong, whether it would be row-ending or something we could remedy. The prospect of potentially abandoning the row due to mechanical failure – something entirely out of our control – filled me with dread. It would have been a bitter pill to swallow.

We worked brilliantly together as a team to turn the boat and get ourselves out of imminent danger, but it was incredibly stressful. Once the initial danger had passed, it was like a pressure valve being released. The stress, fear, exhaustion and tension boiled over as we each handled the emotions in different ways.

With shift patterns completely thrown by the drama, Pip and I retreated into The Hovel to process and recover. When times are tough, it's natural to lean towards those closest to you, and I was so glad to have Pip there as my wingwoman. I also appreciated how much harder those times were for Jo and Lebby, who didn't have a sister on board for support. They continued the rowing shift on deck, and it was a difficult one, with emotions running high and no time or space to decompress as they would have chosen.

It certainly wasn't our finest hour, but it was a testament to our preparation and strength as a crew that it was the first time since starting training that relationships were tested.

Not-So-Happy Christmas

Christmas Day 2021 dawned, bringing a calmer sea-state and a quiet, sombre mood on board. Ocean rowing doesn't stop for Christmas, or give space for licking wounds, and we had a job to do. We had to push aside personal differences and low spirits and focus on our first priority: establishing what had gone wrong with our steering the night before so we could fix it and carry on confidently. The challenge was a welcome distraction, and in the cool light of day, Jo and Pip were able to systematically rule out catastrophic mechanical failure or a freak encounter with marauding flying fish, and put our issues down to a particularly powerful wave sending our autohelm into a tail spin, turning the boat. The relief of knowing that we could carry on was an excellent tonic to the events of the preceding few hours, and once again, confronting and overcoming a challenge filled us with confidence. There was every chance we'd reencounter this issue, but knowing we had the resources to tackle it made all the difference. So often, the fear of the unknown holds us back, but when we can name or see the challenges ahead, we can take the right steps to overcome them.

Heightened emotions had subsided with the Christmas Eve waves, but the reverberations lingered through the day. My default modus operandi is upbeat and jovial, but it's hard to maintain that when it's not felt by those around you, particularly when you're sharing a tiny space. The sombre mood on board only made the pang of missing home and family greater, and there was a lot of inner reflection that day.

Christmas tunes were deployed in an attempt to lift the mood and fill the void that conversation had left. The emotion of Aled Jones' *Walking in the Air* struck a chord with us all, and as the words floated around us, something extraordinary happened. A tiny bird appeared on the wind, a precious gift from Mother Nature. It circled us a few times, dipping over the boat before making another turn. Ridiculous as it may sound, it honestly felt like our guardian angel, sent to lift our spirits and brighten our day. Like small children, we chirped in joy at this unexpected visitor. It was our little ray of light on our day of reflection. That little bird, or another very much like it, subsequently paid us a visit at least once a day, a fleeting but reassuring presence in the vast expanse of the ocean.

Our daily routine of eating, sleeping, rowing and repeating continued, in marked contrast to the Christmas we imagined our families would enjoy at home. We had taken a few small treats and gifts to mark the day, but even these did little to lift the mood. Pip was thwarted by another bout of nausea and couldn't even manage a chunk of my homemade Christmas cake or the special dehydrated Christmas dinner we'd been saving.

It may sound revolting, but the dehydrated roast turkey, complete with roast potatoes, cranberry sauce and pigs in blankets, was the best thing I ate for the entire crossing. Chopped up into tiny cubes, churned together and eaten from a plastic tub with a spoon (the same spoon I used to eat every meal), what it lacked in aesthetics it made up for in taste, or so it seemed to me, at least. It was the culinary highlight of the trip, well worthy of a Michelin star or two. It didn't have to try very hard to win the food prize; we'd been the lucky recipients of the dried food leftover from David's Atlantic row, which was leftover for good reason. My main meals consisted mainly of beef stew, which was so thick and stodgy that it required herculean strength to get through. It was only palatable with a generous dousing of Worcestershire sauce. It was that, or reindeer stew, and even I draw the line somewhere. Lebby, Jo and Pip had the dubious pleasure of chicken korma or lentil dahl for breakfast, noon and night. The bucket got a lot of use, and it's little wonder we all lost so much weight.

With Pip ill and Lebby's palette growing increasingly intolerant, it was left to Jo and me to eat Christmas Dinner for four, doing our bit to keep up the Christmas tradition of gluttonous consumption. Alongside our dehydrated turkey, our other treat was a small packet of Haribo that Pip had thoughtfully given each of us. Haribo was one thing we'd decided not to take but craved, so they were a delight until Mother Nature saw fit to rain on our parade again and swamp my packet with salty water. I persevered for a while, grimacing through the initial salt hit to earn a sweet reward, but in the end had to admit that while salty-sweet may be acceptable for popcorn, it doesn't work with jelly sweets. I hope the fish enjoyed them more than I did.

With uncharacteristically low spirits, I had to brace myself to make satellite phone calls home to my family and parents. I knew they'd be desperate to hear from me, but I didn't want to worry them and risk dampening their day. It was lovely to speak to Paul, Sam, Ben and Grace, and to hear their excited, chattering voices telling me what Father Christmas had bought, full of festive cheer. It was how it should be for children at Christmas, and it brought a smile to my face, knowing they were faring brilliantly without me, and in the best of hands with Paul.

So many people had raised eyebrows at the fact that we were leaving our children over Christmas, and it's something that had preoccupied us as well, but it was a brilliant reminder of how adaptable and resilient children are. So often, the fears or concerns we have on behalf of other people are more a reflection of our fear than others', and if we could only let go of that and be kinder to ourselves, life would be a lot easier. In reality, any concerns I had for my children's happiness were misplaced. They were superstars, making my job of rowing and being away so much easier.

Mum and Dad were celebrating Christmas with my brother James and his family, and they were sat around the table eating Christmas Dinner when I called. It was a fairly chaotic conversation, with eight people all trying to shout things down the phone, and I could hear the emotion – as well as pride – in Dad's voice, as he sent his Christmas blessings. Those conversations were also a reassuring reminder that the world keeps turning, and life continues, regardless of what's happening in our tiny little part of it. I loved speaking to my family and feeling connected to them via the wonders of the satellite phone, but despite the challenges and friction on board, I wouldn't have traded places. I reminded myself of how privileged I was to be experiencing a very different, unique Christmas. There would be many other Christmases to come, when I would take my place around the family table, exchanging gifts around the tree. For now, I was embracing everything about this extraordinary adventure, including the highs and lows of Christmas at sea.

If you go into challenges prepared – with a healthy dose of realism and the expectation that things will be tough, and accepting there will be hard days as well as good – you'll learn, grow and thrive. But go into them assuming it'll be easy, and fearing the hard times, you will likely struggle when they come. I didn't expect the race to be a breeze. If it had been, a big part of me would have been disappointed that it hadn't stretched and pushed me to my limits, that it hadn't tested my physical and mental resilience, that it hadn't been the life-changing experience I'd hoped for, that I hadn't had the full "Atlantic experience." It may sound masochistic, but I wanted it to be hard.

I wanted to experience existential fear, feel the pain and push through it, and know what it's like to complete one of the world's toughest endurance events – the good, the bad and the ugly. Living permanently in your comfort zone will not help you grow, learn or develop as a person, and I've learned that I need to be challenged to feel fulfilled and that I'm making the most of life.

Our Atlantic adventure was like a six-week intensive development exercise, where we learnt some of life's most valuable lessons. Success doesn't come through dodging obstacles or setbacks, but through learning how to embrace them, keep going through them and emerge stronger. We can't control so much of the world around us, and we waste valuable energy if we try, but what we can do is to focus our effort and attention on the things within our control. That's where we can make the biggest difference and determine the outcome. The single biggest thing we can control is how we respond and react to situations and the environment around us. We cannot predict the future or anticipate the details of every situation, but we can learn to predict how we'll react, and how those around us will react, and to draw strength and confidence from our ability to cope with anything life throws at us.

Chapter 10
Ahoy, Land Ahead!

There can't be many events where you feel like you're approaching the end when you still have hundreds of miles and many days left to row.

That's what it feels like when you break the "500 miles to go" barrier. Suddenly, the countdown to the finish line is on, and time starts to slow down. It's a very strange stage in the race because emotionally, you start thinking of the finish and allow yourself to dream about what it will be like to hug your family again. You start trying to pinpoint a date you'll finish and, in our case, set a target. We knew it was unlikely we'd win the women's race, but we wanted to finish in 40 days, and that motivated us to keep the momentum and effort going until the very end.

However, logically, you know you still have a very long way to go. In ocean rowing, disaster can strike at any time. You can't be confident you'll finish the race until you have Antigua firmly in sight. You end up having an internal debate, playing off different voices in your head – the one dreaming of the finish, and the other reigning it in, counselling caution.

Just like at the start of the race, when we'd checked off milestones marking the first "x, y or z," our milestones became the last 500 miles, the last weekend, the last Monday, the last boat clean and so on. Aside from the chart plotter showing our little marker approaching Antigua, nothing else about the seascape around us indicated anything different from the last 35 days – 365 degrees of blue, with nothing breaking up the horizon in any direction.

Conversations on board began to take a different turn, though, with our attention moving to arrangements for the families to fly out to greet us. It's a painful waiting game for supporting families, who are desperate to book their flights and accommodation in Antigua, but are repeatedly advised by Atlantic Campaigns to wait until they get the all-important call to book. That comes around a week from the finish, when they have a good idea of when we'll likely make land. That call is something we all wait anxiously for, too, because it really does signify the beginning of the end. Phone calls to families increase in frequency, as plans are put in place for their impending arrival, accommodation is negotiated, and we put in our duty-free shopping requests. Toiletries are high on the list. Forty days of exercising and sweating, with little more than a few wet wipes for washing, results in an interesting aroma – something we were all immune to, but aware might alarm those still used to their daily showers.

It was an incredibly exciting time, but it was tinged with an underlying and constant sense of anxiety. Before anyone could fly out, they had to pass the dreaded pre-travel COVID tests. Given our experience pre-race, we were taking nothing for granted. The prospect of someone not being able to fly out was almost too much to bear. Visualising our families on the dockside when we finished sustained us for the second half of the race, and it would have been heartbreaking for anyone to have missed out on that.

When we knew when the tests were, we'd make our calls home, hearts in our mouths as we waited for news. One by one, a whoop would emanate from a cabin, followed by a face emerging, beaming with joy and relief and the occasional tear. I still remember making my call and feeling the emotion rising as Paul confirmed they were clear, and the children shouted the news from the back of the car: "Mummy, we're coming to Antigua!"

Pip was the last to get the good news – the night before our families were flying out. We all waited nervously for that call, because we would all have felt the pain and heartbreak, and we didn't want anything to cloud the joy of the finish. Finally, she, too, came out beaming, and we started to relax.

At that point, nostalgia began to creep in. I would happily have paused time for a while to enjoy the incredible experience that was finally coming to an end. I started to reflect on the journey we'd been on – not just on the last 3,000 miles, but on the two years of training leading us up to this point. We'd come so far, overcoming so many seemingly insurmountable hurdles. We'd dug so deep, persevered and maintained our self-belief and determination, ultimately ensuring our success. It had been hard – so hard – but it had also been the most extraordinary experience and extraordinary privilege. I couldn't wait to see my family, but I didn't want the journey to end either.

The penultimate day did feel like time was standing still. The sea had returned to a choppy, heavy state, making rowing hard and uncomfortable, and making it feel like we were going painfully slowly. It was frustrating – we were so close, but still so far. To pass a bit of time, we reminisced about the previous few weeks and how we'd fared. We held an impromptu, very tongue-in-cheek "Mothership Awards," proclaiming "Best Mother" (unanimously Jo), "Worst Mother" (a split decision between Pip and Lebs) and "Mother Most Likely to Need an Inconvenient Poo on Night Shift." The last was the most coveted award, which I had the dubious honour of picking up. I refer back to my diet of stodgy beef stew as the cause.

I clearly remember the final night and counting off the last three night shifts. I savoured those hours on the oars, watching the night sky for the last time and listening to the sound of the waves. As the sun rose for the last time on our incredible adventure, I could hardly believe it would be our final day on board Mrs Nelson. It was a glorious sunny day, with rolling waves and wind aiding our progress towards land, and it was pure joy to row in those conditions, every stroke bringing us closer to our waiting families.

Early that morning, "Pip the Skip" made the call we'd waited two years to make – the "40 miles out" call to Ian Couch, to announce our imminent arrival. I vividly remember her standing in the stern cabin doorway, phone to her ear, speaking to Ian to tell him, "The Mothership is landing." I think we all had tears in our eyes as she made that call.

The last milestone before the finish is sighting land for the first time since losing sight of La Gomera. We spent hours scanning the horizon, trying to make out something other than sea and clouds, until finally, at seven minutes past midday, Pip started jumping up and down on deck, pointing and shouting, "I can see it, I can see Antigua!" It was a joyous moment because now we had something visual to aim for – a target drawing us in and motivating us to push harder.

Over the next few hours, the faint shadow on the horizon grew more defined, and the shape of the island and the hills emerged through the haze. We knew that somewhere on it, our families were enjoying a day of sea and sunshine before heading to English Harbour that evening to welcome us in.

Time to Get Ship-Shape

Our final day was one of the few times when the standard "eat, sleep, row, repeat" routine was broken. We had to get ready for the finish, which meant an array of novel jobs. Off-shifts were focused on tidying and cleaning – both the boat and ourselves.

We'd all fully embraced boat life and, along with it, the freedom of paying scant regard to personal appearance. It's liberating being released from the daily grind of feeling like you need to look presentable. However, as the finish line approached – and with it, the prospect of being seen by other people again, including lots of cameras – we concluded that a nod to some personal grooming was necessary.

Pip and I splurged some of our fresh water for a hair wash. The multi-purpose Dr Bronner's was deployed, and we set to work scrubbing six weeks of grime out of our hair. Complete with Atlantic-breeze blow-dry, we felt pleased with the results and ready to face civilisation again. A certain amount of dysmorphia must have taken hold, though, because on reflection, having seen photo and video evidence, the Dr Bronner's did little to lift the grease.

Jo had the foresight to bring a razor, which we took turns using. It was a great idea in theory, but along with six weeks of leg hair, it precipitated the shedding of six weeks of dead skin cells. I attempted, in vain, to stick them back down with some leftover sun lotion.

The final finishing touch was a small spritz of deodorant, a product we'd dispensed with on day one. Only when I struggled to press the spray button on the can did I realise I'd lost all strength in my left-hand fingers – a side effect of rowing for 12+ hours every day.

With a couple of hours to go, I did something I'd visualised doing so many times during the race. I delved into the depths of The Hovel's furthest-flung hatch to dig out our vacuum-packed, box-fresh finishing kit and presented a set to Lebby, Pip and Jo. It was the icing on the cake for our newly groomed look, and one by one, we took a break from the oars and disappeared into the cabins to wrestle our way into it. Having not worn a bra for six weeks, it was restrictive and oppressive, but we wore them with pride and reappeared on deck to raucous cheers and applause. With our pampering complete, we were ready to face the world again.

The final approach to English Harbour felt painfully slow. Dusk was starting to fall, and every time we rounded a rocky outcrop, we expected to see the harbour entrance – and would be disappointed to see yet more rocky cliffs. Suddenly, we heard voices and saw the lights of a boat approaching through the falling light. It was the media boat, laden with cameras and lights, doing doughnuts around us and the people on board shouting wildly. Having not seen anyone for weeks, it felt very discombobulating being the centre of attention. It spurred us on, and we even found the energy to put in a few hard bursts of rowing for the cameras.

The media boat accompanied us around the final cliff face as English Harbour opened out before us, revealing a dazzling array of lights and sounds. We could pick out the voices of family members cheering from the fort above the harbour; superyachts were blasting their horns, and a few smaller boats had formed an armada to welcome us in.

In the hubbub of noise and activity, we hadn't even realised we'd crossed the finish line – an imaginary line from the fort across the mouth of English Harbour – and the media boat driver had to shout to get our attention and tell us to stop rowing. We looked around in confusion, not quite believing we'd finally done it. That's when we saw Ian Couch on the fort, flare in the air, signalling that we'd crossed the line and completed The World's Toughest Row.

It was Friday, January 21, 2022 – 40 days, 11 hours, and 25 minutes after leaving La Gomera. We let go of our oars and embraced, the emotions flowing: joy, pride, relief, love, respect and excitement. I leant forward and hugged Pip, who had been rowing in the stern seat in front of me. It was a special moment to share as sisters, a strong bond made even stronger by the experience.

We clambered rather ungainly to our feet, stood up and hugged as a crew. This moment I'll remember forever. It was filled with overwhelming gratitude and love for these extraordinary women and pride in what we'd achieved and how we'd achieved it. It was probably the last moment we'd have, just the four of us, to celebrate and appreciate what we'd done before stepping onto land and being swept up by our families.

Next came the razzmatazz of the flares. It's become tradition for each crew to light flares at the finish line, but in the heat of the moment, it's not unusual for crews to inflict serious burns in the process. Staying true to our "Stay Safe" mantra, we took a lot of time to ensure we were holding the flares in the right place and lighting them correctly. I'm sure the media boat crew wondered how on earth we'd made it across the Atlantic when we struggled to light a few flares, but eventually we managed it and stood triumphantly, our flares lighting up the night sky.

It was a magical moment – something I'd visualised so many times since watching David do the same two years before. I remember watching him finish and feeling the tingle of excitement in my spine, wondering what it must be like to stand in that boat, light those flares and achieve something so few people have ever done. Now I knew, and it didn't disappoint. So often in life, reality doesn't match our expectations, but this was not one of those times. The feeling was everything I'd ever imagined and more – the crowning glory on an indescribably brilliant experience.

A Tearful Reunion

When the flares had burned themselves out and we'd safely stowed the remains, we began the slow paddle to the dockside, where our families were waiting. We drank in our surroundings, slowly adjusting to a world that wasn't just sea and sky. The atmosphere was incredible: It felt like the whole of Nelson's Dockyard had come out to see us finish. As we passed one restaurant, they blasted out Queen's *We Are the Champions* and all the diners and staff lined the waterfront to cheer us in. It took us a few moments to realise it was for us. We could see the crowds gathered on the dockside as we approached, their voices growing louder and faces becoming more recognisable with every stroke.

We craned our necks to pick out our families, and I spotted Sam and Ben at the front, wearing their face masks, with Paul holding Grace behind. Their little faces were hard to recognise with the masks, but I could see from their eyes that they were proud, emotional and a little overwhelmed by the whole experience. Then I picked out Mum and Dad, and I could tell how relieved they were.

One by one, we took our final strokes and gently floated into the dockside, to the applause of our family and other supporters. Ian Couch was the first to congratulate us – he'd been the last person we'd spoken to in La Gomera as he pushed us away from our pontoon, and the first we spoke to on arrival in Antigua. As Head Safety Officer, he has the privilege of witnessing every crew's journey, both literally and metaphorically. Over the course of the row, he and his team are there at the end of the phone to offer support, advice and guidance; a reassuring ear or a few words of encouragement. He'd been there to support us through all of our challenges, from signing up in the first place to arriving in Antigua, and we all felt immense gratitude as well as joy when we saw him and were able to say, "We did it."

Ian handed us our "We rowed the Atlantic" banner as we posed for a few final photos on the boat. Then, finally, it was time to take our first tentative, wobbly steps on land. Jo and I clutched each other for support as we stepped off the boat. We were like foals, staggering around on our sea legs, trying to adjust to stable land as we made our way onto the podium for the post-race interview. Carsten, CEO of Atlantic Campaigns, came to me first and asked what my next challenge would be. I laughed it off, saying it would probably be Christmas at home with the family next year. Little did we know how significant that question would be.

After a few more questions, we were ushered through the waiting crowd to a private area, where we were finally reunited with our families. Those hugs said so much; a release of emotion built up over the previous eight weeks. I remember the children's little arms holding on tightly around my neck, wanting to stay as close to me as possible. Then it was Mum and Dad's turn, and it was so special having them both there. Dad wrapped me up in a bear hug, his voice cracking with emotion, so relieved that we'd made it safely and so proud of what his daughters had achieved. He looked exhausted, no doubt in part from his committed dot-watching. It was the first thing he did every morning, the last thing he did every night and often, through the night too.

As we were milling around and catching up, a lady tapped me on the shoulder and gave me a bar of chocolate. She said, "You don't know me, but my husband and I have been following The Mothership, and we think you're amazing. We're so proud of you – thank you for doing what you've done." She and her husband had borrowed a small boat and came out to accompany us on the paddle to the dockside. I remember hearing a man's voice shouting across the water and thinking how much it sounded like Dad. It wasn't; it was a complete stranger who had felt compelled to come out to see us finish.

I forgot about the bar of chocolate and found it again when I unpacked my bags back home. It was then that I noticed there was a handwritten note on the packaging. It read: "I came out here to support Atlantic Buoys. They are my heart, but you girls are my soul." It was one of the most beautiful and generous gestures I think I've ever received – a wonderful reminder of the kindness of strangers. It also made me realise how much we'd impacted not only our own families, but many others, too.

Similar sentiments were echoed throughout our social media channels, and it was humbling to read through all the comments and messages from supporters, many of whom we didn't know. We'd heard the odd snippet through conversations with our families during the race, but seeing them all written down brought home to me how our story and journey had captured the attention of so many.

We'd always said we wanted to inspire our children to dream big and show them that anything is possible, but I'm not sure we believed this would extend further than our families and friends. The effect was so much more than we'd ever hoped for. We were just four ordinary working mums, with a crazy opportunity and enough determination, grit, spirit and support to see it through.

After a couple of hours enjoying the atmosphere of Nelson's Dockyard, it was time for The Mothership to go their separate ways. Saying goodbye to Lebby and Jo was a very odd feeling, having not been more than a couple of metres away from each other for 40 days. But it was family time now, and we headed off to our respective hotels.

Walking through the dockyard to our waiting taxi, Ben wrestled his hand free from mine and instead clung tightly to my wrist. When I asked why, he said, "Mummy, your hand is spiky." I hadn't suffered with blisters, but the constant friction of the oars in my hands had resulted in hardened skin and calluses, which were, as Ben observed, spiky to the touch. It made me smile. It was a small reminder of what we'd done and the impact on our bodies of life at sea.

We had four glorious days relaxing in Antigua, enjoying time together as families and quickly acclimatising to life back on solid ground. Rowers are advised to "decompress" slowly, to process the experience and gradually adjust to real life. However, there's nothing like young children to bring you back down to earth at speed. The minute I was back in the family fold, it was back to being Mummy and everything that entails – relay trips to the toilet, endless rounds of sun cream, nagging to get dressed and clean teeth, anxiously keeping an eye on children in the pool. I wouldn't have wanted it to be any different, though.

Mothering was interspersed with a whirlwind of media interviews. Four midlife mums rowing the Atlantic had captured the attention of media outlets back at home, and we spent a day feeling like celebrities, with TV, radio and press interviews galore. Our phones kept pinging with messages from friends and colleagues who had seen or heard us, and according to several people, it was hard to miss us if you lived in Wales.

Having consumed our body weight in buffet breakfasts, lunches and dinners – and made good inroads into the task of regaining the considerable weight we'd lost – it was with heavy hearts that we boarded the plane back home, to face the cold reality of the British winter and everyday life again.

I wasn't ready to return to normal life – whatever normal is. I wasn't ready to put this unique adventure behind me.

Reflections on an Extraordinary Experience

It's impossible to put into words the experience we'd had – extraordinary, wonderful, challenging, life-changing, life-affirming and so much more. There had been incredible highs and some lows; long spells of serene calmness and moments of abject terror; times when every fibre of my body felt alive and night shifts when every fibre of my body begged me for sleep; all-encompassing laughter and joy and the occasional, uncharacteristic low.

Throughout it all, there was not a moment when I would have wanted to be anywhere else, not a moment when I questioned what I was doing or why I was doing it. For those 40 days, I felt like that little boat, on that vast ocean, with Jo, Lebby and Pip, was precisely where I was meant to be.

Nearly two years in the planning and 40 days at sea, it was the experience of a lifetime, with lessons and memories that will last me a lifetime. The more I digest and reflect on our journey, the more I learn and take from it. It's a privilege and a gift that keeps on giving.

We are all capable of much more than we allow ourselves to believe. Our only limits are the limits we impose on ourselves or the limits other people try to impose on us. If we can silence our inner voices and ignore the naysayers, we open up a world of opportunity.

I've realised that pushing through your comfort zone and testing your limits is not about being fearless but learning to control your fear. It's about learning to use fear as your fuel and motivation to prepare more thoroughly. Fear is a signal that we're challenging ourselves to grow. It's something we should embrace, not avoid.

This journey was the ultimate test of physical and mental resilience. We'd encountered so many challenges and setbacks, but we'd dug deep and realised that however tough it was, we could always give a little bit more and find a way forward. It showed me why we should never, ever give up. Standing on the finish podium, I'd felt invincible. It had proven – beyond any niggling doubts I might have had – that I was tough; a resounding validation of my "nails" superpower. It had sharpened my superpower, taking me to new levels of resilience and confidence in what I could achieve.

Being in a tiny boat, in close confines with teammates – including a sibling – is a nightmare scenario for some people, but I learned that I thrive on connection and relationships. Strengthening my sibling bond with Pip had been an honour, as had forging new, lifelong bonds with Lebby and Jo. I'd learned so much about my own strengths and vulnerabilities, and seen that in the others too.

There's nowhere to hide on an ocean rowing boat. The extreme environment of the Atlantic strips you bare of life's layers, exposing the good and occasionally the not-so-good. We'd all learned to leverage each other's strengths and compensate for each other's weaknesses so that as a crew, we could thrive.

Taking on The World's Toughest Row showed me how much I gain from being challenged and stretched, and how alive that makes me feel. It was the best possible preparation for the challenge that came next.

Chapter 11
My Next Challenge Chose Me

As winter 2022 turned to spring, life did return to normal. Superhero status gradually abated, along with conversations that started, "So, what was it like?" The physical effects of the row diminished as my body bounced back, and within a couple of weeks, I was back on the rowing machine and weight training again. A few physio appointments reversed the muscle wastage in my left hand, and a concerted effort on the nutrition front helped me regain the 10 kg I'd lost with remarkable ease. It had taken the Herculean effort of rowing an ocean to lose 10 kg, and a mere few weeks of enjoying my food to gain it back.

There was just one small niggle which stubbornly refused to go away. My tendency to need an inconvenient poo during night shifts continued, with some mission creep into the daytime too. I brushed it under the carpet for a while, assuming it was the lag effect of the row. However, trips to the bathroom became more frequent, accompanied by uncomfortable cramping. I started to contemplate whether there was more to it than my body's reaction to the physical effort of the row. My dad had suffered from diverticulitis, an uncomfortable condition caused by inflammation of the bowel, for years. So, I concluded it was probably linked.

It was only when I started to notice blood in my poo that I took it more seriously. After a week or so of symptoms continuing, I made an appointment to see my General Practitioner (or GP, as we call our local doctors). I still assumed it wouldn't be anything serious, but in the back of my mind, I remembered reading some social media posts from a fellow Atlantic rower, Ed Smith. Ed's wife, Anna, had tragically died from bowel cancer in her thirties. Ed's crew, Anna Victorious, were rowing to raise awareness and money to support bowel cancer charities, and as part of their campaign, Ed regularly posted about the symptoms.

Sitting opposite my GP, I explained my symptoms, and the young doctor asked if I had any idea what it could be. I told him I suspected something like diverticulitis, given the family history, but also said that I knew my symptoms were consistent with those of bowel cancer. He nodded in agreement, prodded my tummy for a while and told me that although they had to rule out cancer, it was likely to be something less serious. He ordered a blood test and stool sample, and sent me on my way to wait for the results.

Bowel movements tend to be a private matter unless you're on an ocean rowing boat or a young child. Until that point, I'd refrained from sharing the gory details with Paul. However, given the utterance of cancer and the need to send some poo in the post, I decided I should probably give him a heads-up. It was an uncomfortable conversation – as parents of three young children, poo was very familiar territory, but I felt embarrassed explaining my symptoms nonetheless. Paul reacted as I thought he would – brow furrowed, worrying about the cause and probing about the symptoms, making me squirm even more. With my characteristic stoicism, I reassured him all would be well.

I had to wait a couple of weeks to get my results, to allow for the GP to return from annual leave. The surgery receptionist had told me that my case wasn't marked as urgent, and therefore, I could wait for the doctor I'd seen originally to return. This information gave me some comfort. However, when I did speak to the doctor, he informed me that the test results were positive, and he had put me on a two-week pathway for a colonoscopy to do further internal investigation. He reassured me that this test was just to rule out cancer.

Although the prospect of a colonoscopy was not one I relished, I clung to the positives and the doctor's reassurance that cancer was unlikely. So I wasn't overly concerned about the impending procedure. My primary concern was the bowel preparation I'd have to take the day before to "clean out" my bowels, along with the dilemma of whether to have sedation or not. Sedation is highly recommended, as having a camera attached to a tube fed up your bottom and snaking around your insides is uncomfortable, but it comes with the inconvenience of not being able to drive or drink alcohol for 24 hours. My colonoscopy was scheduled for 20 May 2022 – the same day as the World's Toughest Row awards evening in London, something I'd been looking forward to since the race, which would likely involve a tipple or two.

Reluctant to miss out on the celebrations, I decided to forgo the sedation and take the hit on the pain, so that I could then drive to Jo's and meet up with the rest of the crew before the awards event in London.

Friday arrived, and I made my way to the hospital, bracing myself for an uncomfortable hour or so. During my pre-op observations, the nurse remarked on how fit I was and asked what I did. I sheepishly confessed to having recently rowed across the Atlantic, and there was much aahing, oohing, and many questions. Given how fit I was, the nurse reassured me that she was sure everything would be fine.

The endoscopist introduced himself, explained the procedure and asked if I'd be happy for a junior to carry out the colonoscopy. I agreed and hoped that forgoing sedation had not been a reckless idea. With everything set and my hospital gown in place, the nurse wheeled me into the theatre to endure a quick procedure before I could be on my way again and make tracks for London.

If you've never experienced the delights of a colonoscopy, let me explain what happens. You lie on a bed, knees bent, with a large plasma screen in front of you displaying the view from the camera that's being fed into and around your bowel by the endoscopist. It's hardly blockbuster material, but it is interesting insofar as you're unlikely to have ever seen the inside of your bowels before. If you're in any way squeamish, however, I don't recommend it. The procedure started smoothly enough, but after a while, the further the camera penetrated, the more painful it became. I could feel the pressure of the tube as it snaked around, and had to resort to regular slugs of the cocktail of gas and air, which mercifully sent me into temporary oblivion.

Between gas and air highs, I became aware of more activity in the theatre and noted that the lead endoscopist had taken over operating the camera. The doctor's loud voice penetrated through the gas and air fog. "Are you awake?" he said. "Can you hear me?" "Is she awake?" he asked the nurse sitting by my head. Hearing this, I reluctantly abstained from a further slug and told him that I was awake and could hear him. He motioned to the screen in front of me and asked if I could see it and if I knew what it was. Obviously, it was the inside of part of my bowel – but my own bowel is not my usual choice of TV viewing, so I wasn't sure how I was meant to know what I was looking at. He continued, "That's a tumour. You have cancer."

And just like that, in the brief time it took for the endoscopist to say those three words, my world had turned upside down.

I'm all for the direct approach and not beating about the bush, but it was like someone had hit me over the head with a sledgehammer. I was stunned. Speechless. I didn't know what to say, or how I was meant to react. One minute, I'd felt invincible – an ocean rower at the peak of fitness, regaling the nurse with tales of our Atlantic adventure. Next, I was a woman with cancer and a very uncertain future.

Perhaps if I blinked a bit and let the gas and air wear off, those words would somehow disappear, and I wouldn't have to live this nightmare. I could hop off the bed and skip off to my party. But those words didn't go away – they hung in the air, and slowly seeped into my consciousness. I felt dazed, like I was detached from reality and an onlooker in my own story. I was aware that there was a lot of activity around me, and I could hear voices, but the words didn't register, and it was like it was happening to someone else.

Gradually, the haze cleared, and the implications and repercussions of those terrible words started popping up in my thoughts: Paul, the kids, Mum and Dad…. Is it terminal? How do you even begin to process that news in a room full of strangers, lying vulnerable on a bed with a camera and tube still preventing an escape route?

The lovely nurse gently held my hand and asked if I was okay. I nodded meekly, smiling through tearing eyes, not trusting myself to speak, as the endoscopist finished the procedure and removed the tube. The theatre had become a hive of activity, with additional people scurrying around, talking in hushed voices. As the team bustled around me, the nurse asked if there was anyone I'd like to call.

"My husband's in a really important meeting. I can't disturb him," I replied. Ridiculous, I know. Fortunately, she knew better and gently but firmly told me she thought he'd want to know, retrieving my phone from my bag and handing it to me. My hands trembled as I called and left a message asking him to call me back.

Paul's name flashed up on my phone within a few minutes, and I answered.

"Is everything okay?" he asked, worry thinly veiled in his voice.

"Not really," I said. "I have cancer."

"How do you know?" he responded.

"Because the endoscopist has just told me," I replied, a little curtly.

Fortunately, Paul was not far away and dropped everything to hurry to me.

As the team worked away, a wonderfully kind and wise lady – I think she was a senior consultant – approached the bed and explained what would happen next. She inserted a cannula in my hand and offered advice I will always remember and value.

She said, "You're strong. You just need to approach this with the same courage and determination that got you across the Atlantic."

She was right. I had more than proved my mental and physical resilience. I'd lived up to my nails superpower. I could get through this next challenge, too.

I never saw that lovely lady again, and she'll probably never realise how much of an impact her words had, but I'll never forget what she said. She hadn't offered sympathy or pretended to understand how I felt, but she'd reminded me of the strength I had – and would need – to face my new reality.

Words have so much power. They can wound us or be a source of strength and inspiration. Sometimes, we speak without thinking and inadvertently cause pain to other people. Sometimes, we think but don't speak or realise how much those unspoken words might have helped someone. We all have the power to help and heal if we choose our words wisely.

Chapter 12
Keep Calm and Carry On

My Cancer Journey Begins

From the endoscopy theatre, I was taken straight to the CT (Computed Tomography) department for a full-body scan to see if the tumour had spread beyond my bowel. Given how long you normally have to wait for a scan, grateful as I was for the speed, I knew that being rushed through wasn't a good sign.

Lying in the hospital bed, being whisked through the corridors, I felt helpless. I stared blankly ahead, aware of the bustle of hospital life around me but unable to take any of it in. We sped around corners, crashing through doors, leaving the reverberation of swinging doors in our wake. The efficiency of the journey contrasted with the ominous wait for my scan once I'd arrived at the CT department. It was the first time things had really stopped since I'd heard those words, "You have cancer." I didn't know what to think, feel or do. The nurse stayed with me, reassuring me we wouldn't have long to wait, but I couldn't muster the enthusiasm for small talk. Every so often, emotion would rise in my throat – a physical reaction to the news. I'd swallow it away, taking a few deep breaths, staring at a fixed point on the ceiling to steady myself.

I looked around for something to do, struck by the bleakness everywhere. Through the windows of the scanning room, I could hear voices and muffled bleeps. I pondered what my scan might reveal. Would the radiographers be able to see anomalies at the time? Would I be able to read good or bad news on their faces? "I wonder if I'm riddled," kept running through my head. The spaceship-looking white machine across the corridor would be able to see right through me, and would likely hold the answer to the life-or-death question. The reality was as stark as the hospital environment around me.

The scan went as it should, the radiographers giving nothing away. My nurse wheeled me back through the busy hospital corridors through which I'd walked quite happily just a few hours earlier, before cancer had become a part of my life. When we returned to the endoscopy unit, Paul was waiting for me. Tears stung my eyes, but I wanted to be strong – when we'd said goodbye earlier that morning everything was hunky dory. Now, everything was topsy-turvy; life itself was uncertain. Our future was uncertain.

Paul smiled weakly, held my hand and said, "How are you?" There's not much else you can say in those circumstances.

Paul was brilliant. He must have been going through his own emotional turmoil, but he was there for me, and incredibly respectful and thoughtful of what I might want or need, or how I needed him to support me. He asked if I wanted him to do some research for me, look into second opinions and speak to his network of medical professionals. We were very lucky that Paul's job brought him into contact with surgeons and oncologists, so he had people he could speak to. We agreed he'd look into all available options and be my "technical" advisor. It was something he could do to help, and it gave him something to focus on beyond worrying about how I was feeling or the dreaded "what if" scenarios.

After my CT scan, the endoscopist sat down with us to run through the procedure and his report on what he'd found. There it was, written down in black and white – that I had a tumour, with images to prove it. He talked us through the position, size (5 to 6 cm, stretching two-thirds of the way across and around my bowel) and next steps. His debrief contained lots of technical terms and jargon, and it was unintelligible to someone not medically or scientifically trained. Paul asked pertinent questions, with equally confusing responses, while I nodded along, looking between Paul and the oncologist, trying to ascertain what it all meant. I knew that life had taken an unexpected turn, and the future would be very different from anything I could have envisaged that morning. I felt totally out of control of my own life. Two things, however, were clear to me. Firstly, I undisputedly had cancer, and a significantly sized tumour. Secondly, there was no way of knowing at this stage whether it was terminal or treatable – whether I would die from this, or survive it.

The endoscopist had already referred me to the multi-disciplinary colorectal team, who would wait for the results of my scan before agreeing on next steps. The doctor handed us a copy of my report and some generic colorectal cancer information and said one of the nurses would be in touch soon to let me know more.

After the endoscopist left us, I turned to Paul and, in a tiny, wobbly voice, said, "He said it's 5 to 6 cm. Is that big?" I had no idea what 5 to 6 cm in cancer terms represented – whether it was large or small – but Paul's response said it all. He nodded, "Yes, it's big." We both knew what that could mean.

As we walked out of the hospital and into the car park, through the bustling corridors with patients, visitors and staff going about their daily business, where there was the standard scrum for spaces and queues at the ticket machines, it struck me that, while my world had turned upside down, the big, wide world was still turning. It felt like I had a giant, neon sign over my head screaming "cancer." I felt very different to the person who had walked in through the doors a few hours earlier, yet to everyone else, I was just another person going about their daily business. It doesn't matter how cataclysmic a change we face in our individual lives – we're a tiny pawn in the universe, and life goes on around us. Looking around me, I realised that we really don't know what's going on in other people's worlds, behind their smiles or facades of normality.

We drove home in our separate cars, and I imagine we were both lost in our own thoughts. It's hard to process life-changing news like that. How should I be feeling, or thinking? Numb and slightly detached is probably the best way to describe it. It was now a waiting game, and I had to be patient. I had to try not to fear the worst while waiting for the results of the CT scan, which would show whether the cancer had spread beyond my bowel and be a good indication of whether it was terminal or not.

The answer to that question would have such a huge impact on everything and everyone: when, how and what we'd tell people, treatment, family life. My primary thoughts were for my children, who were far too young to go through this, and for my parents. With dad already in the advanced stages of cancer, and knowing full well what the treatment was like, I couldn't bear the thought of burdening them with this huge emotional blow. It's one thing to go through cancer yourself, but another thing entirely to watch a loved one go through it.

With so much uncertainty over my diagnosis, Paul and I decided that we'd wait until we knew more before telling people. I wanted to give people the best news possible, not put them in the same situation that we were in – waiting to find out whether I'd die or not. So, for the moment, we'd both go about daily life as normally as possible.

Tears and Laughter

First things first: that meant packing a bag and driving to Jo's to meet up with The Mothership and then travel into London together for the World's Toughest Row celebration evening. It may seem like a bizarre decision to make, having just heard devastating news, but as the nurse had told me, physically nothing had changed since I woke up that morning. I knew that, in all likelihood, cancer would stop me doing things in the future, and would take things away from me – possibly take everything away – but right now, it didn't have to stop me doing this, and this wasn't something that I could do at any other time. I would have resented the cancer if it had stopped me enjoying a well-earned celebration with my crewmates and the other crews.

It's incredible how you can compartmentalise important things when you need to, and I filed the cancer away in the back of my mind to deal with another day. Of course, it didn't disappear completely, and I found myself contemplating the news occasionally, but I kept it in check. That night was about the row, the community we'd become part of, and nothing else.

We chatted animatedly at Jo's for a while before donning our dresses and getting ready for a night out. Pip and I were sharing a room, and as we were settling ourselves, she casually asked if I'd had a nice morning off. My voice wobbled as I said, "No, not really," hands shaking as I fumbled with the zip of my dress. She looked up, and I could tell she sensed something was wrong. I'm not a drama queen; she knew me well enough to tell by my tone and expression that it was serious. I couldn't hide this from her. I said, "I had a colonoscopy this morning, and they found a tumour. I've got bowel cancer." Seeing Pip's reaction shook me, because until that point, it had been contained in my world with Paul. But hearing it out loud and seeing her devastation at the news hit me hard. There were the obvious questions, which I had no answers to, and we hugged and cried a bit. But after a while, I said, "Please don't cry. I don't want to cry any more. I want to enjoy tonight." So, taking her cue from me, that's what we did.

We put on our makeup, smiled bravely and went out into the night. I'd wanted to tell Jo and Lebby too, because we'd shared so much and were so close – but I knew it wasn't fair. I couldn't tell them before my own family, and I didn't want a dark cloud hanging over their evening. The evening was not about me and my next challenge – it was about celebrating The Mothership and the challenge we'd completed together.

We celebrated our achievements and each other, laughed, drank, danced, and, for the first time since our final day on the ocean, stayed up to watch the sun rise. In many ways, it was magical. I look back on the photos we took that evening and see a strong, fit, happy, smiling woman. It's hard to reconcile that with the reality of my situation.

After not enough sleep, I woke up to face the day – my first day learning to live with a cancer diagnosis. Pip and I hugged tightly before I drove home, so much unsaid in that hug. Although there was much to discuss with Paul, there was no time that day, as we had Ben's 7th birthday party to manage. Trampolining with 20 six- and seven-year-olds wouldn't be my recommended tonic, but parenting doesn't stop for cancer, and we made it through, still smiling bravely.

The next few days felt like living in limbo, waiting for a call from the colorectal nurses to give me the results of my CT scan. I don't think we ever dwelled or felt sorry for ourselves for long, but in our own ways, we got on with living with the news and living life. We had to keep things as normal as possible for the children's sake.

Paul set to work asking scientific questions and finding out about treatments and possible outcomes. I went through the practicalities of notifying work and starting to think about how we'd organise life around treatment. We didn't cry – except for one night when, lying in bed, I turned to Paul and, in a small voice, said, "What if it's terminal? How are we going to tell the kids and my parents?" I knew it would break their hearts, and I couldn't bear to do that to them.

Breaking News

On a Wednesday morning, five days after my colonoscopy, the hospital number flashed up on my phone. It was one of the nurses who had my scan results. It wasn't definitive, but it looked reasonably positive. There were no obvious signs of masses elsewhere, but there were a couple of small blemishes on my liver, which they wanted to get a closer look at. They were fairly confident that they were nothing sinister, so they reassured me as much as possible that the tumour hadn't visibly spread, and I was booked in for an MRI (Magnetic Resonance Imaging) scan later that week to make sure. With that news, and feeling more confident that it would be curable, we decided the time was right to tell our families.

We'd discussed how we'd approach it with our children, agreeing that we needed to be honest but avoid frightening them. Cancer is such a difficult topic to broach with children of different ages, because their understanding and awareness differ. I think for many children, cancer is synonymous with death, and because of this, it is incredibly frightening. They were aware of cancer because they knew that my dad (their Poppa) had cancer, and they knew that Poppa wouldn't get better. We were both worried that they'd assume the worst and think I was going to die, so we had to tread carefully and play it down as much as possible.

One morning after breakfast, while we were all in the kitchen, with me trying to hold my voice as steady as possible, I told them that I had to go to the hospital for an operation to remove a lump in my tummy, and that I'd be gone for a few days but would be back home soon. We'd both thought they'd be inquisitive and ask questions, at which point we were planning to explain that it was cancer, but the only response was, "Okay, can we go and watch TV now, please?" They'd remembered me going into the hospital for a few days for my hip replacement, so the prospect wasn't unnerving for them.

Nevertheless, their blasé reaction took us back somewhat, and we were left floundering around like goldfish, the conversation not having gone as we'd expected. In retrospect, we probably played it down too much, but we didn't want to frighten them by bringing them back in and saying that it was actually serious. So, we left it at that and decided we'd handle the cancer conversation organically when they had questions.

The next conversation was the hardest call I've ever had to make. If I could have avoided it forever and avoided putting Mum and Dad through any more heartache, I would have done so. But it was a conversation I had to have. Sitting in my office with the phone to my ear, my hands felt clammy, and my heart was beating loudly in my chest as I waited for Mum or Dad to pick up the phone. As was usual, Mum answered, and on hearing my voice, said, "Wait a second. I'll put this on speaker phone." I couldn't beat around the bush and said, "I'm afraid I have some bad news. I have bowel cancer." The words hung in the air, silence for a few moments from Mum and Dad, followed by, "Oh, Dids." I could hear the emotion as their voices cracked. I filled them in on more of the details and tried to reassure them that it was likely to be curable and I'd be okay, but I don't think anything can reassure a parent whose child tells them they have cancer. Particularly when you know, from first-hand experience, the treatment journey they're likely to go on.

Mum and Dad had lots of questions, which I did my best to answer, and I thought they'd taken the news well. It was weeks later, after my surgery, that Mum told me how hard the news had hit Dad.

My next call was to my brother, James, who was characteristically understated about the news – shocked, concerned, sympathetic, but mercifully free from emotional outpouring, which I was grateful for. The additional concern that I had for my siblings was the implications for their own propensity to have bowel cancer. Within a few days, James, ever pragmatic, had seen his GP, experienced the delights of a precautionary colonoscopy and received a clean bill of gut health.

Over the next few days, I had to break the news to other family and close friends, including Lebby and Jo. Everyone was shocked, and understandably so. Reactions were consistent: "But how could you? You've just rowed across the Atlantic and you look so well!" On the face of it, I did, but a hidden monster lurked beneath. But despite that, I still felt well, aside from the cramping and additional trips to the toilet.

Ironically, I'd been the most physically robust of our crew, with few niggles and the least tired, managing not to sleep on the oars. Yet throughout the row, and most, if not all, of my training, the tumour had been steadily growing. Looking back, we realised that I did have the initial symptoms of cancer during the second half of the row, when I started getting tummy cramps during night shift, and needing to use the bucket. At the time, we put the change in bowel habits down to the change in our diet (the aforementioned beef stew) and the ordeal that we were putting our bodies through. But of course, with the benefit of hindsight, there was a more sinister reason for it.

My MRI scan confirmed that the minor blemishes on my liver were nothing to worry about, and plans were fixed for surgery a couple of weeks later. My surgeon was a wonderful lady called Kat Baker, who was also a mum and a keen athlete. She told me that she had had abdominal surgery the previous year and returned to triathlons within six months. I was grateful for her words. That information may have been irrelevant to many patients, but to me, it was the reassurance I wanted: that this didn't have to put an end to physical challenges and significant exercise. She also explained that if I had to have chemo, I would likely not lose my hair, and that she would choose a lower abdominal position for the major incision to minimise visible scarring. These vanity points may seem like unnecessary details to communicate when the most important point is the health outcome, but they made a difference for a "young" and active patient like me. She was treating me as an individual, not just as a patient.

Naturally, the kind of person to look on the bright side of life, I was pleased to be classed as "young" again. I don't think that term had been used to describe me for a very long time, and it came as a welcome contrast to the label of "geriatric" during my three pregnancies.

Throughout my treatment, I consider myself lucky to have met some truly wonderful medical professionals at the National Health Service (NHS, the UK's state health service). They may only have been a fleeting part of my life, but whose words and counsel have lingered much longer and whose skills and expertise have saved my life. From the nurse and consultant I met during my colonoscopy to Kat Baker, my surgeon, the team of jolly and kind community nurses, and subsequently, the oncology team of Professor Kerr.

We hear a lot about the troubles of the NHS, but when the chips were down, it was there for me and gave me everything I could have asked for and more – speed, expertise, pragmatism, compassion. I will always be grateful to have won a golden ticket in the lottery of life and been born into an environment blessed with free and comprehensive healthcare.

After the abject uncertainty of my initial cancer diagnosis, and feeling like my world had been smashed to smithereens around me, piece by piece, the jigsaw started to fall into place again, as some of the unknowns became knowns. And so, the plan for my immediate future took shape.

With my new, albeit incomplete and unrecognisable world taking shape, I found a degree of comfort. I knew what I'd have to tackle next, and how I'd tackle it. I had a goal, a deadline, a plan and an army of supporters to help me. This journey wasn't going to be a solo effort; it was going to be a team effort.

Chapter 13
Why *Not* Me?

My surgery was scheduled for Monday, 13 June 2022, three weeks after my colonoscopy and diagnosis. Objectively, it was a swift process from diagnosis to surgery, with a whirlwind of scans, calls and appointments. But it felt like an eternity.

For those three weeks, I knew there was a large, sinister mass in my bowel, growing all the time, and that with each day that passed, there was a greater chance of it spreading beyond my bowel, and a reduced chance of a positive outcome. It was like having a ticking time bomb inside me. Knowing it was there, I just wanted to get rid of it and start the journey to recovery. If I could have reached inside and pulled it out myself, I would have done.

We spent the time putting plans in place for my surgery and making sure we had a support network around us who could help manage the logistics of three children at school and pre-school. We were incredibly lucky to have so many supportive friends and family around to help. I also had to make arrangements to be off work for a few weeks and make sure my team had the support they needed while I was away.

There was nothing normal about everything that was happening in our world, but we did try to keep family life functioning as normally as possible so that the children's world was not turned upside down, either. I carried on exercising, partly because it was a welcome distraction from the cancer and kept me mentally strong, and partly because I knew that keeping my body as fit and strong as possible would help me cope with major surgery and recover quickly. It was a survival instinct for me to continue exercising, but I now know that "prehabilitation" – getting your body in the best physical shape possible before treatment – is an important step that medical professionals recommend.

Inspired by Tragedy

Those few weeks also meant breaking the news to a raft of family and friends, who were understandably shocked given how recently I'd completed the row. There was also the poignant backdrop of the high-profile, tragic story of Dame Deborah James – an unavoidable example of what I might have to face. Around the time of my diagnosis, bowel cancer was getting a lot of coverage in the media because Deborah had very recently announced that she had ceased active treatment for stage 4 bowel cancer and was receiving palliative care at home. It was hard not to draw parallels between us, and when I received my diagnosis, I couldn't help but think about Deborah's journey, her experiences and the impact on her young family.

I watched her last, emotional interview on TV and remember seeing how the cancer had ravaged her body but not her spirit. My heart went out to Deborah and the beautiful young family she was leaving behind. In the days before I knew if mine was curable, it was hard not to wonder whether that would be me and my family soon, too.

Deborah was a beacon of inspiration to me at that time. Even in her final days, she courageously continued with her campaign to raise awareness of the symptoms of bowel cancer, to help other people, like me, seek an earlier diagnosis and not have to go through the immense pain and grief that she and her family suffered.

Awareness saves lives. I owe my future to wonderful people like Deborah, fellow rower Ed and his late wife, Anna, who have selflessly campaigned to raise awareness of symptoms so that others are spared the heartache they have had to endure. A "thank you" seems disproportionate to what they've given me, but I hope that in my own way, I can pay forward to others the debt that I owe them.

A couple of days before my surgery, we enjoyed an early summer's day as a family, pottering around on a friend's boat on the south coast. The children loved the novelty of being on a boat. For Paul and me, it was a welcome break from the practicalities of preparing for surgery, as well as a time to cherish being together as a family before the realities of surgery and recovery took hold. I look back at the photos from that day, and we appear to be a typical, happy and healthy family enjoying a day out. I've often contemplated those images, and I look windswept but glowing – the picture of health. It's far from the image we conjure up when we think of someone with advanced cancer.

It was an early start to get to the Churchill Hospital in Oxford and check in for my surgery. I had specifically chosen to wear a "Rebellious Hope" T-shirt from Dame Deborah's clothing range. Rebellious Hope epitomised Deborah and the way she tackled her illness, and I wanted to draw some of her hope and spirit into my journey as well.

There's a lot of downtime when you're waiting for your operation, and I remember pacing around the room and doing squats to distract myself. I'd taken a book to read, but it was impossible to concentrate. Each time I turned a page, I'd realise I had no idea what I'd just read. The words swam on the pages, as if they had been written in ancient Greek.

Hospital environments are sterile and stark, with stiff, upright chairs, cold floors, perfunctory notices and posters adorning the walls. There's little to raise the spirits, and it's hard to stop yourself thinking about why you're there and what lies in store. I wasn't nervous or scared, but I was on edge, agitated and anxious to get started with the surgery to remove the tumour. I saw the surgery only as a positive. Every moment that passed before surgery, the cancer continued to grow.

It's a very odd feeling, knowing that when you're put to sleep by the anaesthetist, you have cancer, but that when you next gain consciousness, there's a chance you'll be cancer-free. My surgery was a 7.5-hour robotic laparoscopic bowel resection, during which an 11cm section of my bowel, containing the tumour, was removed, together with over 40 lymph nodes, and my bowel was joined back together again. I was very fortunate that, on account of being "young" and of where the tumour was located, I didn't need to have a stoma – an opening in the stomach wall to allow the external collection of faeces.

Lying in my bed after surgery, feeling bruised, battered and very sick but frankly relieved to be alive, I felt compelled to write a Facebook post with a photo of me looking fit and strong with Pip, Lebby and Jo, having just crossed the finishing line of the row in Antigua, alongside a picture of me in the hospital bed with a post-op puffy face and tubes up my nose. It felt like such a stark contrast between the two pictures – the shocking reality that cancer is indiscriminate and can happen to anyone, at any time. I'd completed one of the world's toughest endurance events and felt invincible, yet was oblivious to the unwelcome intruder in my body.

Wistfully remembering my post-row stomach, I tentatively lifted the hospital gown to have a peek at the damage. I'd expected to see dressings and bandages covering the wounds, but instead saw a series of very neat incisions and pen marks making interesting patterns across my tummy, as if marked out for the children to complete a dot-to-dot. While it was horribly swollen and had all the early hallmarks of some severe bruising, it was not the massacre I had imagined.

As I contemplated my post-op body, I wondered whether I was now cancer-free or whether traces of the insidious cells remained somewhere, undetected. From the initial scans, I knew that the tumour had penetrated the bowel wall and may have started to "travel" beyond the bowel into the lymph nodes. Kat Baker told me the operation had gone well. The harvested lymph nodes would be tested for evidence of cancer cells, which would determine the grading of my cancer and any subsequent treatment.

This testing process would take around three weeks, so I had to try to be patient, focus on the positives and recover from surgery, and not worry about the "what if" or "what next" scenarios. Kat's team would call me with the tumour histology results as soon as they had them, and discuss next steps. If cancer cells had spread into my lymph nodes, it would probably mean follow-up chemotherapy, but if the lymph nodes were clear, there may be no further treatment needed.

Cancer is a crash course in learning to cope with uncertainty. To mentally cope with the rollercoaster of diagnosis and treatment, you have to learn how to take each day as it comes and work with the information you have. You have to learn how to control and influence the things that you can in the moment, and be prepared to adapt – mentally and physically – as you go along.

The Road to Recovery

Recovery was reasonably straightforward and quick. The second night was painful and sleepless, as the hard-core drugs had worn off, and I struggled to find the right balance of pain medication. However, on the whole, I bounced back quickly and was on my feet, shuffling around the ward the day after surgery. As I pulled my trolley of medical gizmos behind me and did laps of the ward corridors, I became increasingly aware that I was in the minority. Most of the other patients on the ward seemed to be confined to their beds, and as the physiotherapist explained, often lacked the strength in their upper bodies to push themselves up to a sitting position, let alone climb the proverbial mountain of getting out of bed.

Far from feeling sorry for myself and indulging in the downward spiral of "why me" thoughts, I felt so lucky to be in the position that I was in, with age on my side, an Atlantic row under my belt, and with it, the strength and fitness to recover quickly. "Why *not* me?" was genuinely my attitude. I knew I was in a much better position than most of the patients around me, and it motivated me to work harder on my rehabilitation and return home quickly to a more comfortable environment.

Seeing my progress, the doctors even gave me a "pass" to leave the ward and venture outside into the warm June sunshine. I bought a cold drink from the hospital shop and found a bench in the garden, where I sat, face turned up towards the sun like a sunflower. Fresh air and sunshine do wonders for my soul, and I could almost feel them healing me, physically and psychologically.

I was desperate to get back home to Paul and the children and knew that the key to getting there was to show that I was physically strong enough and able to cope independently. I treated my rehab a bit like training for the row, seeing it as a challenge and always aiming to go beyond expectations. If the physio suggested three laps of the ward, I'd give myself a target of four or five. And that was how, after just three days, I was given the green light to pack my bags and go home.

Wearing my "Rebellious Hope" T-shirt, clutching my green hospital bag of medication, and walking away from the hospital holding Paul's hand felt like a major milestone in my cancer journey. I felt like I was walking away from my tumour.

I was far from the sprightly woman who had walked into the hospital, but the wounds would heal, and as far as we could tell, the tumour had gone. It was short-term pain for long-term gain.

Mum was waiting for us at home when we arrived and enveloped me in a hug and love that only mothers can give. I was so grateful to have her there, but it hadn't been an easy decision for her to come. Dad's journey with cancer had taken a turn for the worse, and he was struggling to heal after a lengthy surgery to remove several secondary tumours. I wanted her to stay with Dad because I had Paul and the children to look after me, but Dad was adamant that she should come. I appreciate that, as parents, we have an insatiable need to care for our children, regardless of their age. While Dad couldn't make the journey from Wales to be with me, he made sure that Mum did. He wanted Mum to see me with her own eyes and be able to reassure him that I was okay. A phone call wasn't going to cut the mustard.

Pip and James, along with their families, rallied around to help and be with Dad, so that Mum could spend a couple of days with me. Although the circumstances that brought it about were far from ideal, having that time with Dad was special for them both and has given them memories they cherish.

General advice after surgery like mine is to aim to walk for 45 minutes by the time you reach six weeks post-surgery. I recovered quickly and felt strong and well. Within a couple of weeks, I was able to walk for 90 minutes, finding comfort and enjoyment in being outside in nature and exercising. Abdominal surgery limited the kind of movement I could do, so walking was the limit of my physical endeavours. I knew it was doing me good, both physically and psychologically. Moving around and being outdoors in the fresh air helped my body heal and keep me strong, and in the process, it also kept me mentally strong. I felt that if I could still walk at a decent pace, covering significant distances, then surely I was going to be ok and beat the cancer. My daily walks became a significant part of my recovery, healing both body and mind.

At a time when daily life looked nothing like it had before and when there was so much about my situation that I couldn't control, exercise became something that I could. It was my way of clinging on to an element of normality in a very abnormal world.

Earlier in the year, Pip and I were invited to be guests of honour at our old school's Speech Day and Leavers' Service in early July, where we were asked to give an inspiring speech to the children and parents. I can still remember being in the audience at Speech Days when I was a pupil and listening to some extraordinarily inspiring speakers, so I couldn't quite believe that Pip and I had been asked to speak. However, with my surgery less than three weeks before Speech Day, it looked unlikely that I'd be able to do it.

As the days went by following surgery, and I became stronger and stronger, I started to focus on Speech Day as a milestone to reach, a day when I would be mentally and physically strong enough to stand up in front of several hundred people and share our story. It was something I wanted to do and also felt I needed to do. I wanted the opportunity to stand proudly alongside my sister and tell our story. I wanted to inspire the next generation to dream big, and show them that ordinary people – like us, like them – can achieve extraordinary things. I needed to take the opportunity to stand up there and tell the whole story, the twist in the tale, to pay forward the gift of awareness that I had been so fortunate to have. While I knew it would be difficult to do, and it would also be difficult for Pip, and for Mum and Dad, who would be in the audience, I felt it was important that I shared that element of the story. It was a way for me to help raise awareness of bowel cancer and potentially help someone else in the future.

A couple of days before Speech Day, I heard the familiar rustling of the post landing in the hallway, and as I stooped down to collect it, I saw that one of the letters was stamped "Oncology Department." I walked through to the kitchen where Paul was standing, showed him the envelope and said, "It looks like I'll be having chemo then." Sure enough, the envelope contained an appointment letter for an oncology consultation the following week. I knew that could only mean one thing – the cancer hadn't been entirely contained in the bowel and had spread to some other cells.

A little investigation led to a very apologetic call from the colorectal nursing team, informing me that I should have received a call to explain the results of the tumour histology before the letter arrived. As we'd deduced, cancer cells had been found in some of the lymph nodes, which meant my cancer was stage 3, and the recommended course of action would be chemotherapy to "mop up" any remaining cancer cells. I had known this was a possibility, but seeing it written in black and white was a stark reminder that the cancer was in charge here, not me. It was also a realisation of how advanced my cancer had become. The idea that I'd be back at work at the end of the summer, with cancer behind me, was now blown out of the water. My next challenge would be the perils of chemotherapy.

Finding out I'd need chemo felt like the aftershock of an earthquake. Just as I was starting to feel better, I was faced with a second wave of turmoil and upheaval – an extended period of feeling worse, to hopefully make me better. It was another prolonged uncertainty and disruption to life plans. It signified that my cancer was worse than we'd thought. While that is obviously not good news, a part of me welcomed the additional treatment. I knew the treatment would make me feel horrible, far worse than the cancer itself had ever done, and I knew I would be in it for the long haul. But it was described as a "belt and braces" approach to hit the cancer hard, and that suited me. I wanted to throw everything at the cancer, leaving no sliver of opportunity for it to remain lurking somewhere, unseen. I was prepared for any level of misery if it meant a better chance of a healthy future.

I was also curious to know what chemotherapy was really like. It would give me a better understanding and empathy for what Dad had gone through. Chemo is so synonymous with cancer; it conjures up images of people sitting around the perimeter of a hospital ward, attached to drips for hours on end. People in varying stages of hair loss, with faces pale and gaunt. I'd been reassured that I wouldn't lose my hair, but how would it affect me? Would my superpower protect me? I was about to find out.

Sharing My Story

Speech Day came, and I was excited to get dressed up and meet the Headmistress, Governors and other dignitaries. Pip and I felt like imposters, giggling nervously as we filed in as part of the "platform party" and took our seats on the stage in front of hundreds of pupils, teachers and parents, some of whom had been pupils alongside us decades before. I looked out at the sea of expectant faces and couldn't quite believe that I was there. We were just two ordinary mums who had jumped at an opportunity to go on a mid-life adventure. I hoped they weren't expecting superheroes.

Pip and I stood shoulder to shoulder, recounting some of our tales and lessons that we hoped would inspire the audience. We concluded our speech by talking about "the next challenge" – one of the questions all ocean rowers are asked, and the first question I was asked when I completed the race. As I talked openly about my diagnosis, surgery and impending chemotherapy, there was pin-drop silence, and I could see people dabbing their eyes, including my mum and dad. Pip's voice faltered as she wrapped up our speech, and I put my arm around her. I often think that, hard as cancer or any serious illness is for the patient, it can be harder for your loved ones, who carry such a burden of anxiety and a feeling of helplessness.

During the reception after the ceremony, numerous people came up to me to express their appreciation and share how much they were inspired by hearing our story. Several people talked about their own experience of cancer, and how seeing me and hearing me had given them a different perspective. One parent, Victoria Taylor, sent us a note afterwards to express her thanks. I cried when I read it. She wrote:

> Today, you have armed my girls with the most powerful of tools they could acquire. They have come away talking about moving on in life by thinking of the reasons as to why they should do something rather than the reasons why not. Added to that, they have seen and heard that there is greatness in each one of us and that it's not all about academics, sports, drama, etc. It's about championing your inner self. Seeing how two sisters

adore and respect each other, and are friends, gives me hope.

You two are incredible women, and everything you have said and demonstrated has impacted all of us there today. You represent everything I want my girls to be and feel. Thank you for your humour, humility and generosity of spirit.

When we decided to do the row, we'd said we wanted to inspire our children and other children. It was something that united us as a crew, but I don't think we ever fully appreciated the impact we could have. Hearing from some of the pupils, parents and teachers made me realise what a privilege it is to be able to share our story and inspire others. Although I had no idea of how significant that realisation would be, or what it would lead to, at the time, the experience of sharing our story at my old school was the first building block of a new career.

Dad was exhausted after the ceremony. We'd gathered at Pip and David's for lunch afterwards, and usually the life and soul of the party, he was uncharacteristically quiet, spending almost the entire time resting in an armchair. Always one to make light of hardship, he had earlier joked about the benefits of being granted a disabled parking space alongside the marquee, which would give him VIP status. Seeing him then, I felt the truth behind his words keenly.

I wanted to enjoy the occasion, having our families together, but gnawing away, never far from the surface, was a deep concern for Dad – an overwhelming sadness to see cancer stealing the life from him. I sat next to him as he held my hand tightly and told me how proud he was of me for being so open about my cancer. He said these words in a hoarse whisper, because a secondary tumour had started to impact his speech. It broke my heart to see and hear how the cancer was ravaging him, and that I'd had to put him through the additional worry of my illness, the stage 3 diagnosis compounding his fear.

Mum and Dad left after a short while, so Dad could rest properly, and Pip and I helped them out to the car, looping our arms around each other and watching in heavy silence as they drove away.

We couldn't have known, but that was the last time I would see Dad walk.

Chapter 14
Life Can Be Cruel

The Healing Power of Nature

July 2022 was a quiet month, spent gradually building my strength and stamina to prepare my body for the next challenge of chemotherapy. There were parallels with July 2021, which was a month of intensive water and land-based training as we built our strength and stamina ahead of the race. The goals, while very different, were equally a foray into uncharted territory: endurance events that would challenge my physical and mental resilience. They were both inherently difficult to predict – from the duration, to the conditions, risks, physical and mental consequences and even the outcomes.

I found immense comfort and peace in nature. While my abdominal surgery meant I couldn't run or weight-train, I replaced my usual regime with long, brisk walks around the countryside, which helped me regain fitness. Through the additional time I had outside and at home, I developed a new interest in flora and fauna, observing things I'd never really taken an interest in or had time for before. I'd spend ages just looking at our little patch of garden every day, willing it to morph into something worthy of the Chelsea Flower Show – sometimes pottering with planting or weeding. Watching the fruits of my labour develop was a surprising source of joy; watching them subsequently perish, less so. I am not green-fingered, but I enjoyed the distraction and unusual sense of purpose it gave me. There is so much unexpected joy to be found in the small things in life that, so often, we take for granted.

After my daily walk and garden contemplation, I'd look forward to the ritual of morning coffee and toast with Paul. It became a highlight of my days, and still is now. I'd regale him with an account of my morning's work, proudly show him the latest development in the garden or lament the latest plant victim to have withered in my care, much to his amusement. The local garden centre experienced a boom that summer.

My rehabilitation also allowed me to spend more undivided time with the children, something I now cherish and don't take for granted. It doesn't mean I don't have all the usual frustrations and challenges of parenting, and I'm far from a perfect parent, but I truly value that time. Not having to juggle work with the rest of my life, I was able to pick them up from school every day and enjoy the summer with them, free from the usual guilt and worry that I was neglecting either work or family, or both.

Alongside recovering from surgery and regaining strength, treatment plans and logistics were put in place for chemotherapy. Paul and I met with Professor Anne Kerr, my oncologist. There are many things in life we can aspire to, but having an oncologist is not one of them. I remember being acutely aware the first time I said the words "my oncologist." Much like uttering the words "I have cancer," it's something you never expect or want to say. Having an oncologist puts you in an unenviable – and sadly, not niche – club. A necessary evil club.

I was grateful to have Paul with me when I met Professor Kerr for the first time. There is so much medical terminology involved in a cancer diagnosis and treatment that I'm sure it bamboozles most patients, including me. Having someone there with a more advanced understanding of medical terminology than most, who could listen, ask pertinent questions and later act as a translator and sounding board, was incredibly reassuring. Professor Kerr explained the histology of my tumour and results in detail, illustrating the "grading" of the cancer and the implications of that from a treatment perspective. She was transparent with the facts but empathetic, and didn't shy away from talking about my prognosis and chance of recurrence. I listened, strangely detached, as she quoted percentages – not able to compute that these black-and-white numbers represented the likelihood of the cancer returning and life-changing consequences. She talked about chemotherapy being a choice. But really, it didn't feel like there was a choice.

As a wife and a mother to three young children, staying alive to be there for them was my number one priority, and I would have done anything to increase my chance of a cancer-free future. Without further treatment, the chance of the cancer returning was 40%. With chemotherapy, the chance of recurrence is reduced to 27%. There wasn't a decision to make. It had to be chemotherapy.

Hearing those numbers, I was shocked at how significant the chance of recurrence was, even with chemotherapy. Somewhere deep in my psyche, I still felt like an invincible ocean rower, like cancer had been a blip in an otherwise healthy life. The statistics told a different story. Chemotherapy wasn't going to be the golden bullet to dispatch cancer for good. But I'll take 27% over 40% any day – and flipping it on its head, 73% chance of staying healthy is a much more reassuring way of interpreting the numbers.

Cancer recovery is a case of playing the long game. There's no quick fix, hit-it-hard-and-move-on approach. For five years after treatment, I'd be at risk of – and monitored for – recurrence. And even then, there are no guarantees that it won't return. There wouldn't be a line drawn in the sand, or a big declaration of "all clear." It would be five years of hoping and praying I stay healthy, punctuated by the mental rollercoaster of tests and scans, during which time the risk of recurrence gradually decreases. It's the ultimate test of mental resilience.

Coming to Terms With a Heartbreaking Reality

Towards the end of July, we'd planned a large family get-together for my mum's side of the family. Mum is one of five siblings, and over time, as more and more offspring arrived on the scene, we'd outgrown anyone's house and gathered in a village hall. It's always a happy, boisterous affair, with children running wild and tables laden with enough food to feed an army. Mum and Dad loved these family occasions and, having hosted them for many years, were part of the scaffolding that held the occasions together.

I was looking forward to seeing them both before a short family holiday in Suffolk and then starting chemo, but a few days before the get-together, Dad developed a chest infection and was admitted to the hospital. He was still upbeat about coming, but as the day grew closer, it became evident that he wasn't well enough to travel, and he and Mum made the decision not to come. We all felt their absence acutely. As the eldest of the siblings, Mum had always worn the mantle of matriarch, and Dad, the patriarch. It felt like the central piece of the jigsaw was missing, and conversation naturally turned to how he was.

Following Dad's lead, Pip and I were positive, but a conversation with Annabelle, one of Mum's sisters, floored us both. Annabelle was a doctor and the family's medical sounding board. She and Mum spoke regularly, and she gently told Pip and me that, given Dad's cancer and steady deterioration over recent weeks, she didn't think he'd have long left.

Carrying bowls of half-eaten food and the children's paraphernalia back to the car, I struggled to hold back the tears, not wanting to break down in front of everyone, particularly the children. It felt like a heavy, dark cloud had descended, and I couldn't find a way out.

Looking back, I realise we'd probably been burying our heads in the sand. Objectively, Dad's health had been steadily deteriorating since before the row. We'd had a long time to get used to the idea that Dad's cancer was terminal, but he'd kept defying his prognosis and responding so well to treatment. And he was so determined and positive about bouncing back that I think we all believed that would be the case. He'd never stopped making plans for the future or living life to the full.

Our hope that he would rally and keep going gave us a false sense of security, as it was a much happier perspective than considering the alternative.

After the family gathering, Paul, the children and I travelled to Suffolk to house- and pet-sit for our great friends, Sian and Ali. We couldn't travel abroad because of my treatment, but their beautiful house provided a much-needed family break before I embarked on the unknown rollercoaster ride of chemo.

I wanted to return to Wales to see Mum and Dad, but Pip reassured me that she would be there and would keep me updated. I knew the situation was grave, but still, a glimmer of hope remained. As long as Dad was receiving treatment, there was hope, and I clung to it.

Midway through the week, I was watching the children and Paul in the pool and saw Mum's name flash up on my phone. A sixth sense told me immediately that it was bad news. Tears cascaded down my cheeks as Mum told me that Dad was not well enough to have any further treatment, and that he was coming home to receive end-of-life care. It was news I'd expected and dreaded. Confirmation that, after a valiant and generally healthy four years, Dad's journey with cancer was finally coming to an end.

I stood in the kitchen for several minutes, silent, trying to process the news that had broken my heart. I stared into the distance, seeing nothing through my tears, a numbness preventing me from moving. An excited squeal from Grace finally permeated my consciousness, and I saw her tearing across the lawn, pink towel streaming behind her. I brushed the tears from my face as I went outside to meet her, looking to the sky and taking a few deep breaths, smiling at her through my pain. Paul quickly followed, and one look at my face told him everything he needed to know.

We returned from Suffolk, and I repacked a bag before driving to Mum and Dad's, unsure of what to expect when I arrived. Pip, who lived locally, had kept me updated on Dad's condition, but it was still a shock to see him so visibly weaker than when I'd seen him at Speech Day earlier in the month. He slept for significant periods of the day, and when he was awake, his breathing was laboured and conversation tired him quickly. Despite this, he retained his spirit, humour and courage.

It was heart-wrenching to see Dad steadily decline over the next few days, but it was also a special, peaceful time. We spent hours just sitting with him, sometimes reading or chatting. Sometimes we would just sit and listen to the birds singing and feel the warm summer breeze through the windows. Mum had moved a table up to their bedroom so we could eat our meals there. Although he wasn't able to be active in conversations, he enjoyed listening to us chatting around the table, as we had all done so happily for so many years. Now and then, he'd quip something from the bed to let it be known he was listening and still had an opinion. His interjections would invariably bring a smile to our faces, and sometimes laughter. His body may have lost its strength, but his spirit shone brightly still.

Accepting that Dad didn't have long left, Paul and the children also came to visit. It was an opportunity for them all to say their goodbyes to their beloved Poppa. He wasn't strong enough to see them for long, but I know he appreciated seeing their faces and having the opportunity to say goodbye himself. It was so hard to watch, knowing that it was the last time they would see and cuddle this wonderful person, who had been such a huge influence in their early childhood and had adored seeing them grow up.

After a couple of weeks with Mum and Dad in Wales, I reluctantly had to return home to Oxford to start chemo. Dad was asleep and peaceful most of the time, and when it was time for me to leave, he was sleeping. I gently kissed him goodbye, told him I loved him and drove home. I didn't know that would be the last time I'd see him alive.

Getting to Grips With Chemotherapy

The children were excited to have me home, wrapping me in their little arms and immediately drawing me back into family life. They knew I was sad, and although they couldn't express it in words, I could see they were trying to make me feel better. The following morning, we went fruit picking, dodging wasps and gorging on sun-warmed strawberries and raspberries. It was a simple summer holiday activity as a family – a brief taste of normality amidst the turbulence that surrounded it.

It was an important time with the children before life was disrupted again by the unknown world of chemotherapy.

Early that afternoon, we left the children with Paul's parents, Chris and Barry. We then made our way to the Churchill Hospital, the specialist cancer treatment hospital in Oxford, for my first infusion of chemotherapy.

Walking through the corridors to the chemotherapy centre, we passed lots of other patients. Some were pulling trolleys along with them, and many bore the hallmarks of typical cancer patients – gaunt faces, hair loss or bright scarves tied around their heads. I wondered if I would soon look like that, too.

I didn't know what to expect as we walked into the chemotherapy ward, but I was surprised to see it looking exactly as you see them on television. I don't know why that surprised me, but it was disconcertingly familiar, down to the maroon of the high-backed, faux-leather chairs stationed at intervals around the perimeter, to the trolleys alongside them, suspending the bags of fluids, emitting an array of bleeps and flashes as nurses strode purposefully in and out.

We were shown to my maroon chair and settled in for the next few hours. I felt conspicuous, sitting there surrounded by so much obvious illness, when I looked so well. I was suntanned, fit and strong, a relative youngster compared to most patients. I felt like a fraud.

As a "newbie" to chemotherapy, there was a lot of preliminary and administrative work to go through before I even got to the infusion part. With COVID restrictions still in place, Paul was allowed to join me for my first infusion, but from then on, I would be on my own. I was glad he was there to serve as a second pair of ears, listening to the overwhelming volume of information that was given to us, so that he was also aware of what we might expect from the next few months of treatment. While I was the patient, we were a team. We had to navigate the consequences together. If there were pieces to pick up, he'd be the one bearing the weight.

First, I was given a goody bag of medication with a detailed rundown of what to take, why and when. I quipped to Paul that I'd need one of those tablet boxes to sort my tablets by day. Then it was an explanation of a terrifyingly long list of potential side effects and what to do if I experienced any of them. It was sobering listening to the cautionary words as I realised how much chemotherapy put me at risk of so many different ailments, from infection and sickness to heart failure.

There was also the challenge of dealing with an uncertain timeframe. I was due to have six rounds of chemo, each lasting three weeks, but the timings were dependent on my body recovering sufficiently from the previous round to be able to tolerate the next round. So, while it may be over in 18 weeks, it could be longer. I couldn't pin my hopes on being finished by a certain date, because it would set me up for disappointment. I just had to take each round – each day, even – as it came, and know that slowly but surely, I'd get through.

Once the lengthy explanations were complete and the anti-sickness drugs had had some time to take effect, I was finally hooked up to the chemo machine. The little bag of clear fluid looks so innocuous, but looks can be deceiving. You know it's a bag of poison that will not only kill the cancer cells, but also kill your healthy cells too. Drop by drop, you watch the poison transfer from the bag into your body, and it's a waiting game – waiting to feel something different. But what it is, you don't know. It could be any, or many, of the long list of side effects you're told about.

You have to get comfortable playing the waiting game with chemo. My infusion was two hours, plus the preamble – a long time for me to be sitting around inactive, but relatively short compared to some treatments. I'd brought along various activities – colouring, books, podcasts, and, of course, Paul. It was also a time to think, reflect and just observe everything around me. Each cycle, I'd look around the room at the other patients and wonder what their story was. What particular strain of the terrible disease had brought them here? How far through were they? What did their future look like?

It always made me grateful to be in the position I was in – young(ish), fit and strong, and better prepared to withstand the effects of the treatment than most. Most patients were considerably older than I, and many looked frail. When I thought about what they were going through and how hard it must be on their bodies, it made me feel so lucky to be going through it at this stage in my life.

On the flip side, one thing that surprised me was how many young people there were, too – lives turned upside down by cancer when they're only just getting going. I was lucky to have had my children before cancer came knocking, but so many people face not only the pain of treatment, but also the lasting damage it does to your body, including fertility.

Sitting in that room, as a cancer patient and surrounded by cancer patients, also made me think about Dad and how much he'd had to endure over the last four years.

Finally, I had a little glimpse into what he and Mum must have gone through. He never complained – he was stoic throughout, and so positive and grateful to have the option of treatment to extend his life as long as possible. I imagined him and Mum sat in these chairs, holding hands, chatting, probably striking up conversation with other patients and making the nurses laugh. Dad had a wonderful ability to put his own troubles aside to help others, wherever he was.

I didn't have to wait long during my first infusion to feel the effects. Very quickly, I felt like ice was flowing through my veins, starting at the point of infusion and spreading like tentacles throughout my body. It was unpleasant rather than painful, and a sign that the drugs were taking effect.

Part of me had expected to sail through treatment and get away lightly with side effects. That's the nails part of my identity kicking in, along with my optimistic outlook. But there was also an element of me that welcomed the side effects, because they reassured me that the drugs were doing something and improving my chances of a cancer-free future – no pain, no gain, as they say.

With the final drops of chemo dispensed and armed with a pharmacy of drugs, Paul and I were relieved to walk out of the ward with my first infusion under my belt. It was a beautiful summer afternoon, and although the air was warm, my fingers, feet and lips tingled, like icy pins and needles. If that was the amuse-bouche of chemotherapy, we waited to see what the next course would bring and when it would arrive.

Getting back home was like stepping back into the real world, and I enjoyed the distraction of the bustle of family life. There's nothing like small children to keep your feet firmly planted on the ground and worries at bay.

I called Mum to let her know that I was home and had safely completed the first infusion, and I could hear the relief in her voice. She said that Dad was much the same, sleeping most of the time and generally peaceful. I agreed to drive back to see them the following day, once I had a better idea of how my body would react to the chemo and felt safe to drive.

For now, all was as well as it could be. Aside from the unusual intolerance to anything remotely cold, I felt fine and was glad to have started the next stage of treatment. It was another significant milestone that I could tick off.

In some ways, tackling cancer was like tackling the Atlantic row, or any other big undertaking. It was a huge challenge, with a defined goal, but an uncertain and very long timeframe. Pinning all your hopes and sense of achievement on the outcome is demoralising, so you have to break it down into smaller steps and find milestones that you can realistically achieve and celebrate. Those milestones serve as motivation to stay positive and keep moving forward. By focusing on the next step, it doesn't feel so overwhelming.

It was also about learning to live in the present, rather than dwelling on the past or longing for the future. Bobbing around on a little boat in the Atlantic, I truly came to appreciate what it meant to just *be* and find comfort and joy in the small things. The same was true of cancer. There was no point in looking back and wondering if somehow I could have avoided it, and I couldn't know what the future might bring or put my life on hold until some time in the future when I could leave behind treatment and monitoring. It was about living each day as it came and being grateful for everything I had in the moment.

Chapter 15
Losing an Anchor

It was Tuesday, August 9th, 2022, the morning after my first infusion of chemo. I woke and lay in bed for a few moments, wiggling each part of my body and assessing how I was feeling. Happily, beyond the tingling, there seemed to be no further side effects yet. I knew they would take a while longer to kick in, but I was relieved to be feeling reasonably normal.

I had planned to spend the morning with the children at home and then drive back to Mum and Dad's in Wales.

With a fridge full of berries from the previous morning's picking, we set to work making jam. The kids ate almost as many berries as went in the pan, and it was a chaotic, happy time – a welcome slice of normality in my topsy-turvy world.

As the fruit bubbled away, Pip called. My heart lurched as I reached for my phone, a now familiar sense of foreboding catching in my throat. "Is everything okay?" I asked.

"The nurses are here. Dad's breathing has changed, and they don't think he has long left. I think you'd better come back now."

I grabbed my bag and stash of medicine, hastily gave Paul some instructions on how to make jam and leapt into the car for the two-hour drive to Wales.

It was a long journey, and the miles seemed to go painfully slowly. I willed it to go more quickly, desperate to be by Dad's side, but I also wanted time to stand still. I didn't want to face what I knew was coming.

As I turned into Mum and Dad's driveway, I noticed that only Mum's car was parked there. I knew James wasn't there because he was touring Europe with his family, and Dad had been adamant that he shouldn't come back. But where was Pip? And the nurses? I didn't need an answer to know what it meant.

With a heavy heart and trembling hands, I walked into the kitchen to see Mum making a cup of tea. She looked over, and with tears in her eyes, said, "Oh, darling, I'm sorry, Dad died this morning." We hugged for a long time – there was nothing much either of us could say.

Dad had died peacefully, with Mum and Pip holding his hands, not long after Pip had called me earlier that morning.

I couldn't have made it back in time, and they knew it wasn't right to tell me before I left and risk me driving while processing the news.

The evening before, after I'd spoken to Mum to let her know I was feeling okay after chemo, Pip had told Dad that I was safely through my first infusion. He'd nodded gently, acknowledging the news, and it was the last time he was conscious and visibly responsive. I like to think the news gave him some comfort and the reassurance he needed to rest in peace.

Finding Strength in Community

The next few days passed in a haze of grief. There was a constant stream of people coming through the house to offer condolences or conduct some of the endless administration that follows a death.

I felt like I was in a daze – desperately sad, mentally and physically exhausted, yet unable to sleep. I'd crawl into bed at night, hoping sleep would bring respite. But instead, with no distractions and only my thoughts for company, when I turned out the light and closed my eyes, the tears would flow. I'd toss and turn, staring at the ceiling and blinking back tears to avoid morning panda eyes, but each time I managed to turn off the tap, another thought would send them flowing again.

Nausea meant mealtimes were a futile exercise in pushing food around the plate, breathing deeply to settle my stomach and trying to will myself to eat something to keep my energy levels up.

In the midst of it all, I had a treatment follow-up call from one of the chemo nurses to find out how I had responded to my first round of chemotherapy. She ran through a series of standard questions inquiring about my physical and mental health.

"Are you feeling low?" she asked.

"Yes, but my dad's just died," I responded.

"Are you feeling sick?" she asked.

"Yes, but that may be the grief," I replied.

"Are you sleeping okay?"

"No, because when I close my eyes, the tears flow."

It was impossible to tell whether my symptoms were a result of the chemo, grief or a mixture of both. I suspect it was the double-whammy effect of potent drugs combined with the loss of a parent. Life hadn't just given me one lemon – it had sent a grove-full tumbling down on me.

It doesn't matter what life throws at you – somehow, you find a way of dealing with it, because what other choice is there?

In those times, you truly come to appreciate the people around you who are there for you with so much love and support. I count myself lucky to have such an amazing network of friends and family who helped me through both my cancer and losing Dad.

There's often not much they can do practically to help, but simply reading their thoughtful messages and knowing they were thinking of us helped.

When you experience challenges with other people, you have a deep understanding of what they're going through. This shared emotion can bring you closer together and strengthen bonds. Sharing your pain and vulnerability helps you navigate a path through, and together, you can be stronger.

Sometimes you'll need a helping hand or a shoulder to cry on, and sometimes you'll be the one who can offer that support. When you find a way to support others, too, you gain strength from having that purpose. It keeps you going because other people need you.

Losing a parent is hard, but I think losing your life partner of more than 50 years is harder, and Mum needed us. We supported each other during that time, sharing the heartache of losing Dad, dealing with the administration and funeral arrangements together, crying together, reminiscing together and sometimes laughing together.

Mum was an inspiration. She is so strong, capable and stoic. Despite her grief, she found the strength to support us through ours, and together we found a way through the toughest of times.

Paul was, and continues to be, my rock, stabilising and supporting me through whatever comes our way. We tackled cancer as a team, both of us motivated not only by supporting each other but by supporting the children. They were our reason to keep positive, to keep going and to keep life as stable as possible.

Through Dad's final weeks and after he died, Paul was the mainstay who kept our family running, enabling me to spend precious time with Mum and Dad. He was the emotional and practical support for us all, helping the children through their first experience of death.

Dad had been a pillar of the local community – actively involved in the local council as both a councillor and Deputy Leader for many years, as well as a non-stipendiary priest, leading services in some of the local churches. He was loved and respected by many, and we expected a big turnout for his funeral. To enable as many people as possible to attend, we delayed the funeral until the start of September, to minimise the clash with the summer holiday exodus.

Alongside funeral planning, I also had to schedule my next round of chemotherapy. It's important, particularly as a new patient, to monitor how your body reacts to the drugs. So I had a mid-cycle telephone appointment with one of the oncology consultants to assess how I was feeling and plan the next round. During the call, the consultant asked if I had any particular side effects, and I reported that I felt tight-chested when running.

There was a short pause as she digested this. Evidently, not many people run during chemo, and this was the first time she had encountered this feedback. As chemo can cause heart complications, she suggested that my symptoms might be related to the particular drugs I was on, and therefore, it would be prudent to review the cocktail for my next round.

Fortunately, she didn't tell me to stop running – that was a lifeline for me – but as a consequence, she recommended a different combination of drugs, which would mean a longer, 48-hour infusion. For the first round, I would need to be an inpatient, so that they could insert a PICC line (peripherally inserted central catheter) to administer the drugs and closely monitor my heart.

We agreed to a short delay in starting my next round so that we could have Dad's funeral without the risk of further complications. It was going to be hard enough to get through as it was without worrying about potential side effects. I also wanted to take the children to school for the first day of the new school year. It was Grace's first day of primary school, and that was a milestone I didn't want to miss.

Finding the Light in Darkness

On 2nd September 2022, we said our final goodbyes to Dad, burying him in a beautiful spot on the edge of Wolvesnewton Churchyard, overlooking glorious Welsh countryside. Wolvesnewton had been our family home for many years, and since his ordination in 2017, Dad had taken many of the services in the church.

Hundreds of family, friends, former and current colleagues came to the funeral, and it was wonderful and humbling to hear and read so many accounts of how he had touched people's lives. I hope Dad knew how much he meant to his family, friends and colleagues.

James, Pip and I stood shoulder to shoulder to give his eulogy. It was one of the hardest things I've ever had to do, but it was a privilege and an honour to stand alongside my siblings, recounting tales from his colourful past and paying Dad that final respect.

It would have been easy to find reasons not to stand up and give the eulogy. But just because something is hard doesn't mean we shouldn't do it. We had to ask ourselves, "How will I feel if I don't do it?" and "How will I feel if I *do*?" We knew it was the right thing to do – for Dad, for Mum and for each other – and together, that helped us to find the strength and courage to do it.

It was undeniably tough to lose Dad to cancer while going through my treatment. It felt like life had dealt me – had dealt all of us – a viciously cruel hand. When the grief cloud settled, my thoughts would spiral. Why did this have to happen? And why did it have to happen now? Did we miss something years before that could have saved Dad? Was there a treatment somewhere that we could have tried?

But Dad's words penetrated the bleakness, bringing me back, if not to harmony, then to acceptance. Whenever we faced challenging times, Dad would say, "Everything happens for a reason." His wisdom helped me see things in a different light.

Even in those darkest of days, I learned to be grateful that my illness had given me the opportunity and privilege to spend those last precious weeks with Dad, and then have the time with Mum to support her through the difficult early weeks of learning to live without him.

Without my own cancer, I'd have been knee-deep in work and on a time-clock of carer or bereavement leave, feeling guilty about not being in work and feeling like I had to return to work too soon. Thanks to my illness, I didn't have to think about work, and that was a blessing.

I don't believe in living with regrets, because it doesn't serve anyone and can't change anything. But I will always be sorry that cancer and chemo prevented me from being with Dad when he took his final breath. That's the only part of my journey that I'd rewrite.

I truly believe that every cloud has a silver lining somewhere. It might not be immediately obvious, and it might take time to appreciate it. But if you look hard enough, for long enough, you'll find a glimmer of light.

Chapter 16
The Rollercoaster of Chemotherapy

The start of a new school year always heralds much excitement and activity, even more so when you're starting school for the first time, like Grace. Our house was a bustle of labelling and laying out uniforms, packing pencil cases and bags, polishing shoes and chattering about seeing friends and new teachers.

Grace was delighted to be joining her big brothers at "big school," with grand intentions of learning to read, write and play catch-up. I love the first morning of school every September – the frenzy of getting three children ready for school and desperately trying to keep them looking neat and tidy, in some semblance of order for the ceremonial "first day of school" photo. For once, the children bounce out of bed and into their uniforms, gobble down breakfast and are eager to make the short drive to school to see their friends.

That morning was also tinged with the nervous anticipation of my next instalment of chemo and a few days in hospital. We all trooped off to school, and while Sam and Grace trotted happily into their classrooms, Ben was more reluctant, clinging to me, refusing to let me go. It was out of character, as he's normally such an outgoing, brave and independent little boy. He's also the most emotional of the three, and I knew he was reacting to both Dad's death and my own illness. I feel for parents who have to go through this every day – it goes against all your parental instincts to prise little hands off you and leave them somewhere they don't want to be.

It's so hard trying to explain death and cancer to children. In Ben's mind, Poppa had cancer, went into hospital and now wasn't here any more. Mummy also has cancer, and is going into hospital. It's logical to be frightened.

Although I'd already experienced a chemo ward once, this time was very different. Whereas the outpatient chemo ward was strangely familiar, having seen it on TV so many times, the inpatient cancer ward was an alien environment. It was set up like a typical hospital ward, with shared rooms and some individual side rooms. Most patients looked bedridden, clearly very unwell. I, on the other hand, still looked fit and healthy – a curious anomaly.

At check-in, the nurse told me that she expected to see me doing laps of the ward, skipping up and down the stairs. I think they'd been briefed on why I was there.

I was glad to be given one of the side rooms, which had its own bathroom, ample space and privacy. The first task was a procedure to insert a PICC line. Having done my research, I wasn't looking forward to this. It's like a semi-permanent cannula, with a line running through your veins from your arm to somewhere deep in your chest. It means the drugs can be distributed more directly. Because it stays in place, it makes it easier to hook up and disconnect different infusions, minimising the damage inflicted by endless needles.

The procedure was mercifully less painful than I'd imagined, with the preamble far worse than the reality. After some testing and flushing, I was hooked up to the first of two infusions. I'd have a 2-hour infusion, followed by a 48-hour infusion. The latter was fed from a "balloon pump," which I'd have to carry around with me in a little shoulder bag. As accessories go, it was hardly Chanel.

After the initial flurry of activity, I was left to my own devices, with my first infusion dripping away. Usually upbeat, I felt bleak. It was hard to be positive, being thrust back into a cancer environment so soon after Dad's funeral, with only strangers around, knowing it was only a matter of time before the physical effects of the chemo kicked in.

Cue Mum. While a cancer ward was probably the last place she wanted to be, she came anyway and was the chink of light I was missing. Walking onto that ward to support a daughter, having so recently done the same thing for a husband, must have taken all her resolve and strength. But I needed her, we all needed her – and I think Mum needed to be needed, to fill the vacuum left in the aftermath of the funeral.

Seeing Mum so strong was the inspiration I needed to pull myself together and find my positivity again.

If you can find a purpose to cling to, whatever that may be, it will give you the strength and motivation to pick yourself up when all you feel like doing is curling up in a ball and giving life a wide berth.

I did my best to fill the time while the infusions trickled in, but I lack the patience to sit around doing nothing. I paced around the ward, making endless cups of tea just to occupy myself, and found a little respite in the small, broadly concrete "garden" off the ward, where I could appreciate the final rays of summer. I even experimented with a few physical exercises, curious to see whether my heart would react and how much mobility the PICC line allowed. I was determined that this latest inconvenience wouldn't get in the way of staying fit, and I would find a way to work around it.

Desperate to leave the hospital, I'd packed my bags ready to be discharged after my second long night, but my eagerness was not rewarded. A steady stream of nurses came along to check my balloon pump to assess progress, and in the end, they concluded that the line had kinked and the infusion had stopped. Left with no choice, I was incarcerated for a third night to allow the infusion to finish and give the nurses confidence that I wasn't going to keel over with a heart attack.

Navigating the Waves of Chemo

I was finally free to leave early the following morning, and as I walked away from the hospital to my car, I felt like I was walking through clouds. Everything seemed to be in slow motion – or at least everything in my brain was in slow motion. Chemo brain fog had descended, and it was wholly disconcerting.

I drove home slowly, unnerved by the odd sensation, and was grateful that Mum was there to look after me when I arrived. I had no energy or inclination to do anything other than lie on the sofa and doze. I didn't feel particularly sick or ill in other ways, but I was physically and mentally exhausted – lacklustre, tired to the bone. I'm sure three nights in hospital with interrupted sleep had contributed to the fatigue, but the chemo effect was definitely at play. It was an all-encompassing level of exhaustion I'd never experienced before – not even through years of breastfeeding through the night or the 40 days of sleep-deprived rowing.

The exhaustion, combined with a general physical and mental malaise, continued for the next few days and was something I simply had to get used to over the subsequent rounds of chemo. When I stopped to think about it logically, it made perfect sense. My body was being poisoned. It was bound to have an effect.

Completing the row had made me feel invincible. Chemo had put me firmly in my place.

I braced myself for the tidal wave of excitement and chaos that would descend when the children came home from school, and I mustered the energy to be there at the door when they arrived, full of smiles and hugs.

Mum and Paul tried to shield me from the full force of the children's enthusiasm, but I was determined to put on a brave face for them and do as much as possible with them. It was important to me that they didn't worry, and that their lives weren't tarnished by it any more than they had to be.

Sam and Grace were keen to see the PICC line, and their squeamish curiosity amused me as they squealed at the sight of the strange, flappy thing sticking out of my arm. Ben, on the other hand, held back, hiding behind the door, afraid to look. Throughout my chemo, he hated seeing the PICC line, and whenever he noticed it poking out from under the "cuff" I usually wore to protect it, he'd plead, "Put it away, Mummy!"

The PICC line was the only visible sign that I was ill, and for Ben, it was a daily reminder of the cancer and of all the frightening associations he had with it.

By bedtime, I was shattered, my energy levels depleted. It was all I could do to crawl to my bed after tucking the kids into theirs.

Having Mum at home for the next few days was a godsend. She did the heavy lifting with the school run and mealtimes, and was generally there for company and to make sure I was looking after myself. It also gave Paul the opportunity to travel to the office in London for work after a summer of inevitable disruption.

The fog and exhaustion gradually lifted, and it was a relief to feel something close to normal again. Normal meant exercising, and I resumed running and gentle sessions on my rowing machine.

My PICC line limited my range of movement, but where there's a will, there's a way. I found ways around it and worked out what I could and couldn't do.

The line was restrictive, so upper body strength training wasn't advised. As it was an external line into my chest, it carried a reasonable risk of infection, so I couldn't swim or have my arm submerged in water for any length of time. It also caught on clothing, and I had to be careful not to knock it. But running and machine rowing were achievable.

The PICC line dressing had to be changed, the wound cleaned, and the line "flushed" regularly, so for the duration of my chemo, I was under the care of the wonderful local community nursing team.

On the morning of my first scheduled visit from one of the nurses, I returned home from a run, hot and sweaty, to find the nurse had arrived early. I chased her car up the drive, breathlessly apologising for my state, but she was delighted. She told me that one of the big challenges in her role is getting her patients to be active. I joked that she'd find the challenge with me would be getting me to rest.

With round two of chemo safely navigated, and my heart happier with the new blend of drugs, I settled into my new routine and we found a way to manage family life around the hospital trips, nurse visits and periods of total wipeout. I had to find a way of working with the chemo, not against it. It wasn't a short-term game – we were in it for the long haul.

Six rounds would take around three months to complete. But one of the many challenges is the uncertainty around timings and duration, and I knew it was a fool's game to pin my hopes on finishing by a specific date. I mentally built in a contingency, targeting Christmas as the deadline to be finished and well on the road to feeling like myself again.

While every round brought a slightly different mix of side effects, and the effects were typically cumulative over time, we could reasonably predict how I'd be feeling during each three-week cycle. Week one would start with a hospital visit and infusion one, followed by infusion two over the next couple of days at home. Aside from the cold, tingling sensation and some mild brain fog, the first few days were tolerable enough, with exhaustion setting in by midweek and lasting for a few days. By the middle of the second week, I was starting to bounce back, usually having a good final week before it started all over again.

People often ask how I coped with chemo as a mother of young children. In some respects, it did make it more physically challenging, but they were an absolute blessing. They gave me a reason to be positive, to be active and to keep going – a reason to get out of bed every day, to get dressed and not wallow in self-pity.

There are also the practicalities of family life, which meant that I had to keep going. Children aged 5, 7 and 9 require physical and emotional care. The demands of life didn't stop just because I was having treatment.

Paul had borne the brunt of running the household while I recovered from surgery and couldn't drive, and then again around Dad's death when I spent time in Wales. That was, of course, on top of two months flying solo while I took a little jaunt across the Atlantic. It inevitably compromised his ability to work standard days and, particularly, to travel to an office, but it's not a lasting solution. Working late into the night to make up time and keep on top of a busy workload isn't sustainable. As soon as I could, and as often as my treatment allowed, I picked up more of the family responsibilities.

Paul's employer and colleagues were a brilliant source of support throughout, understanding of the situation and providing moral, professional, and practical support for us. I might have been the one who was ill, but the ramifications for Paul, as chief carer, were huge. It's at times like those that you truly appreciate the value of a supportive, people-first work environment. Anyone can print words on a page about well-being and duty of care, and deliver the contractual requirements outlined in policies, but the real measure is in what you experience when you need it. It's about being human first – showing you value, care and understand.

When I reflect on 2022, and the burden it placed on Paul, our wedding vows come to mind: "for better or worse." I like to think he generally gets an excellent measure of the "better" (as do I), but 2022 seemed to hand out a lion's share of the "worse."

At the end of October, I arrived at the Churchill Hospital eager to get started on my final round of chemo. It was a huge milestone – hopefully the last time I'd take my seat in the maroon chair and be hooked up to the now familiar chemo machines.

I'd taken my anti-sickness medication in anticipation. I was ready for the infusion when one of the nurses told me that my white blood cell count wasn't sufficient to be able to tolerate any more chemo safely. I'd have to return a few days later and try again. It was a mental blow, but not unexpected. I knew delays and setbacks were all part of the chemo journey, and so I was prepared for the disappointment and stoic about the delay. It was a minor detour in the path, not a major roadblock.

The invisible effect of chemo on your body accumulates over time, as it struggles to process the drugs and recover between cycles. My body had just had enough for the moment and needed more time.

The following week, I returned, this time less confident about whether I'd be able to have my final round. Fortunately, although my white blood cells were far from abundant, there were enough to allow the infusion to proceed. The end of the chemo road was in sight.

I had to return to hospital a few days later to have my PICC line removed – a remarkable procedure that was over in seconds, with the flick of a skilled nurse's wrist. And with that, she told me I was free to go, to leave the ward that was now so familiar, and hopefully never return.

I thanked the nurse, picked up my bag and walked out. There was no drama, razzmatazz, fuss or even acknowledgement that I had completed chemo. I hesitated as I walked past the reception desk, looking over my shoulder and half expecting a nurse to be hurrying after me, with a form to sign, or perhaps even a bell to ring. But nothing.

It was a moment that was so deeply momentous for me, yet so unremarkable to those who see patients coming and going, day in and day out.

Having expected to feel elated, it was an anticlimax. As I emerged from the bowels of the hospital into the chilly November afternoon, passing patients still in the thick of treatment, I reflected on this.

My treatment journey may be over for the moment, but for thousands of others, it wasn't. I was lucky.

It was a lesson in perspective. We may feel completely consumed by something, but however large, significant or insurmountable it seems in our lives, it may pass unnoticed by others – and there are always others facing something bigger.

It was also a lesson in finding comfort and joy within oneself, rather than relying on external validation. It was a momentous moment for me and for those close to me, and that was something worth celebrating. I didn't need anyone else to give me a gold star or ring a bell for me.

As I pulled out of the car park, leaving hospital life behind me, I blinked back a few tears – tears of relief and gratitude to have made it to this stage, when so many, like Dad, don't.

Chapter 17
Finding My Light at the End of the Tunnel

I was totally unprepared for how I would feel finishing chemotherapy.

It was like falling off a cliff.

Once the initial malaise from the final round had subsided, I thought I'd skip off into the next chapter of my life, feeling like the weight of the world had been lifted off my shoulders.

I thought I'd be full of joy, hope and relief.

Instead, I felt like I was in freefall, the unlikely comfort blanket of cancer treatment taken away from me.

Since my diagnosis, everything had been about proactively treating my cancer, hitting it hard with a ferocious combination of surgery to remove the mass, then round after round of chemo to eradicate any remaining cells. While the doctors and drugs attacked cancer from one direction, I exercised, ate well, slept well and did everything I could to help my body fight it organically.

Suddenly, it felt like my recovery was in the lap of the cancer gods, with the reassurance of proactive treatment taken away from me. Either the cancer would return or it wouldn't, and aside from looking after my physical well-being myself, I wasn't doing anything to stop it from coming back.

I just had to wait and hope. It's not a short wait, either. It's five long years of being monitored to see if it rears its head again. Even after that, there's still a chance. Cancer isn't something you can ever put in the past.

Naively, I also thought I'd bounce back to full health and fitness quickly. I looked fine, and day to day, I felt fine, but the invisible damage ran deep. The lingering side effects knocked the wind out of my sails. I stubbornly pushed through and launched myself back into gym work, but it was hard graft to build up my strength. Even after treatment had finished, new side effects emerged. Weeks later I started noticing tingling in my toes, and the soles of my feet became sensitive, like I'd walked on burning sand. It was just another, potentially permanent, gift from the chemo gods.

Onwards and Upwards

I had a choice to make. I could let the uncertainty, the fear of "what if" and the anxiety get the better of me. I could let the threat of cancer hang like a dark cloud over the next few years. Or, I could choose to accept and adapt to the circumstances and get on with the job of living life.

I wasn't going to let cancer define the next five years.

If there's one thing I've learned, it's that life is short. We should live it.

We started with a holiday in the sun to celebrate the end of treatment and my being able to travel again. I'm a big believer in celebrating the milestones, and this was a big one. After everything that had happened over the previous six months, which had been so hard on Paul and the children, too, it was what we all needed. It was a chance to relax, rest and recuperate as a family, and it was a chance to mark a line in the sand – the end of one chapter and the start of the next.

We came home to a big family Christmas with Mum, Pip, James and the families. It was busy and chaotic, but a very large piece was missing: Dad.

12 months before, when Pip and I had celebrated Christmas amid the Atlantic, away from our families, we dreamed of the

next Christmas at home, visualising what it would be like. We couldn't have foreseen what was to come, or how it would turn our worlds upside down.

When you lose someone you love, the first Christmas – like the first birthday, anniversary or any other significant occasion – is hard. Dad's death was still raw, and we all felt his absence deeply. He loved nothing more than a big, bustling Christmas, with his family all around him. Christmas was a union of two things that meant so much to him: family and faith.

We had the big, bustling Christmas, but the sparkle was missing.

Life doesn't return to normal after cancer treatment ends, because you move into the next challenge: being monitored. For me, it's a five-year period, punctuated by blood tests, scans and colonoscopies to check for signs of recurrence. The likelihood of recurrence is highest during the first two to three years after treatment. In my case, a 27% chance of cancer returning somewhere. Professor Kerr told me to have a party in year three, and a big party in year five.

Five years is a long time in any context. It's hard to imagine getting to the end and wondering what the path might look like in between. The only way to approach it is to keep positive about the outcome and accept that there will be twists and turns along the way. You have to tackle it day by day, week by week, scan by scan, knowing that each day that you get through healthy is a good day, and a day closer to those parties.

This period can feel a bit like being on an emotional rollercoaster. As your next scan or test approaches, "scanxiety" builds until you get the all-clear, then you can relax for a while before bracing yourself for the next ascent.

As someone blessed with a glass-half-full approach to life, I know I have a reasonable chance of recurrence at 27%, but I choose to focus on the 73% instead. I'm much more likely to remain healthy, or at least, cancer-free, than I am to find cancer knocking at the door again. I'm now in the middle of my five years, and the journey is more of a gentle undulation than a rollercoaster.

Colonoscopies aren't my idea of a fun day out, but I don't dread the scans and tests, and I don't feel anxiety getting the better of me. (Paul may disagree.) It's reassuring to me to know that I'm being checked regularly, and I take the view that if something is found, it will be caught early and can be treated.

Five years of constant worry about the what-if scenario and putting life plans on hold would be miserable for everyone. It's much more comfortable to assume the best and stride forward through life with purpose.

I have had to accept some changes, though, and learn to adapt to them. I've always dismissed minor aches and pains, assuming they're just a part of life and will go away in time, occasionally to my peril. My hip niggles are a case in point. But through various life experiences, from childbirth to hip replacement and cancer, I've concluded that I have an unusually high pain threshold, and my body is a master at disguising and hiding issues.

I have to learn to find my inner hypochondriac and be vigilant to the slightest ailments, in case they're something sinister, rather than just the unfortunate consequence of approaching my half-century. It's not easy, and I'm still a work in progress.

Paul is helping. He does most of the worrying for both of us. And although I roll my eyes when he gives me that "look" after I confess to a niggle, I'm grateful that he's looking out for me. We're an excellent team. He's also become my barometer for anything relating to the children's health. They'd have to be carrying a severed limb or be at death's door before I resort to intervention or allow them to skip a day of school. Consequently, they have almost unblemished school attendance records.

Our ability to adapt is critical to tackling challenges and navigating change. As Jamie, Pip's eldest son, used to cite when he was a small and very articulate child, "Dinosaurs became extinct because they failed to adapt to their changing environment."

My children may think I'm a dinosaur in age, and after 40 days at sea, I was probably a little scaly, but I hope that's where the resemblance ends.

Cancer can have a devastating impact on lives, and it can take so much away from us. For too many people, it takes everything away. But if we look beyond the initial horror, it can also give us so much, and it doesn't have to stop us chasing dreams and making plans. For me, it's a bump in the road, not the end of the road.

Cancer has taught me to appreciate the things that really matter and find joy in the everyday things that we so often take for granted: reading bedtime stories to the children, morning coffee and toast with Paul, spring flowers emerging from their wintery beds, family, friends, health, the motivation and ability to keep fit and active, memories from the past, opportunities in the present and the prospect of a future.

It has taught me that life is short, so I should live it and be grateful for it. Every. Single. Day.

We never know what's around the corner, so don't wait for tomorrow; live today. But that doesn't mean live it at one hundred miles an hour and cram so much into it that you burn out. It's about not letting life happen to you but living with intention. Seizing opportunities and creating opportunities, but also knowing when to say "no." Being "all in" or "not in," but not wavering in between.

It's given me a new purpose and a drive in life and work. I know how fortunate I am to be able to share my story when others don't get the chance to tell theirs. I was given the gift of awareness, and I hope that by sharing my experience, I can pay this forward and help someone else in the future.

Somebody once asked me if I would change anything about the recent past, and it's something I've often contemplated.

If I could, I would rewrite Dad's story and give him more time to live the life he loved with Mum.

I would have made it back to Wales to be with Dad when he died.

But I wouldn't change anything else.

Our past and our experiences shape who we are today. The lessons we learn equip us for what lies ahead.

We can't change the past any more than we can predict the future, but by accepting and embracing the past, with all its inevitable highs and lows, we can face the future with confidence, curiosity and courage.

Epilogue

I'm now midway through my five years, and so far, so good. Party season is approaching, if I heed Professor Kerr's advice.

I'm also heeding my own advice. My experiences have given me the self-belief, self-confidence and self-worth to know that I can achieve anything I set my mind to. They've encouraged me to take control of my career, connect with my purpose and find new opportunities and adventures. I will mark the three-year milestone since my cancer diagnosis in the foothills of the mighty Mount Everest, tackling the world's highest marathon.

The mindset and approach that I used to guide me across the Atlantic and then through cancer have since helped me through work turmoil, redundancy and a new career as a professional speaker. It's a huge privilege to connect my purpose and passion, sharing my experiences and the lessons I've learned from both my personal and professional life to help other people and businesses thrive.

Turn back time five years, and I had no inkling that life was about to take me on a journey that I couldn't possibly have envisaged.

It's been a journey of breathtaking heights and inky dark depths, glory and misery, successes and failures, laughter and tears. It's been a journey of discovery, and I've learned so much about myself and others. I've learned about the human spirit's ability to endure, its generosity in helping others, the strength we gain in numbers and how to navigate the never-ending waves of life and emerge smiling, whatever the weather.

We can bury our heads in books, take all the courses under the sun and have an alphabet of letters after our names, but the school of life provides the best education. It's usually easier to hunker down in the safety of our comfort blanket than step out into the unknown and challenge ourselves to do something different. However, when we push ourselves outside our comfort zone, we learn, develop new skills and gain a deeper understanding of ourselves, our values and the world around us. We fill our toolboxes with resources that will help us in life and enable us to become more resilient.

Sometimes, we can choose to be challenged; sometimes, life chooses to challenge us. Either way, the key to success and thriving is to approach each challenge we face with the right mindset, with the right people around us and with a commitment to work hard.

The path of least resistance is not always the right path to take. To achieve our goals and dreams, we have to expect to face stormy seas. We have to be prepared to put the effort in to get the results we want.

With the right mindset and hard work, ordinary people, like you and me, can achieve extraordinary things. We all have those voices telling us we can't do something. But if we can learn to silence those voices and use our fears as fuel, we can persevere through setbacks and darkness, emerging stronger. We do it for ourselves, and we do it for the people we love.

There is greatness in every one of us. You will have different strengths from me. We're not better, not worse, just different. Embrace what makes you different and harness your superpower to help you navigate your challenges and discover your own version of extraordinary. Tell yourself, "I can, and I will." Because we *all* can.

Whatever oceans we're crossing in life, there will be storms we have to face.

We can choose to let each storm stop us in our tracks or push us off course, or we can choose to lift ourselves up and be stronger than the storm.

We all have that choice.

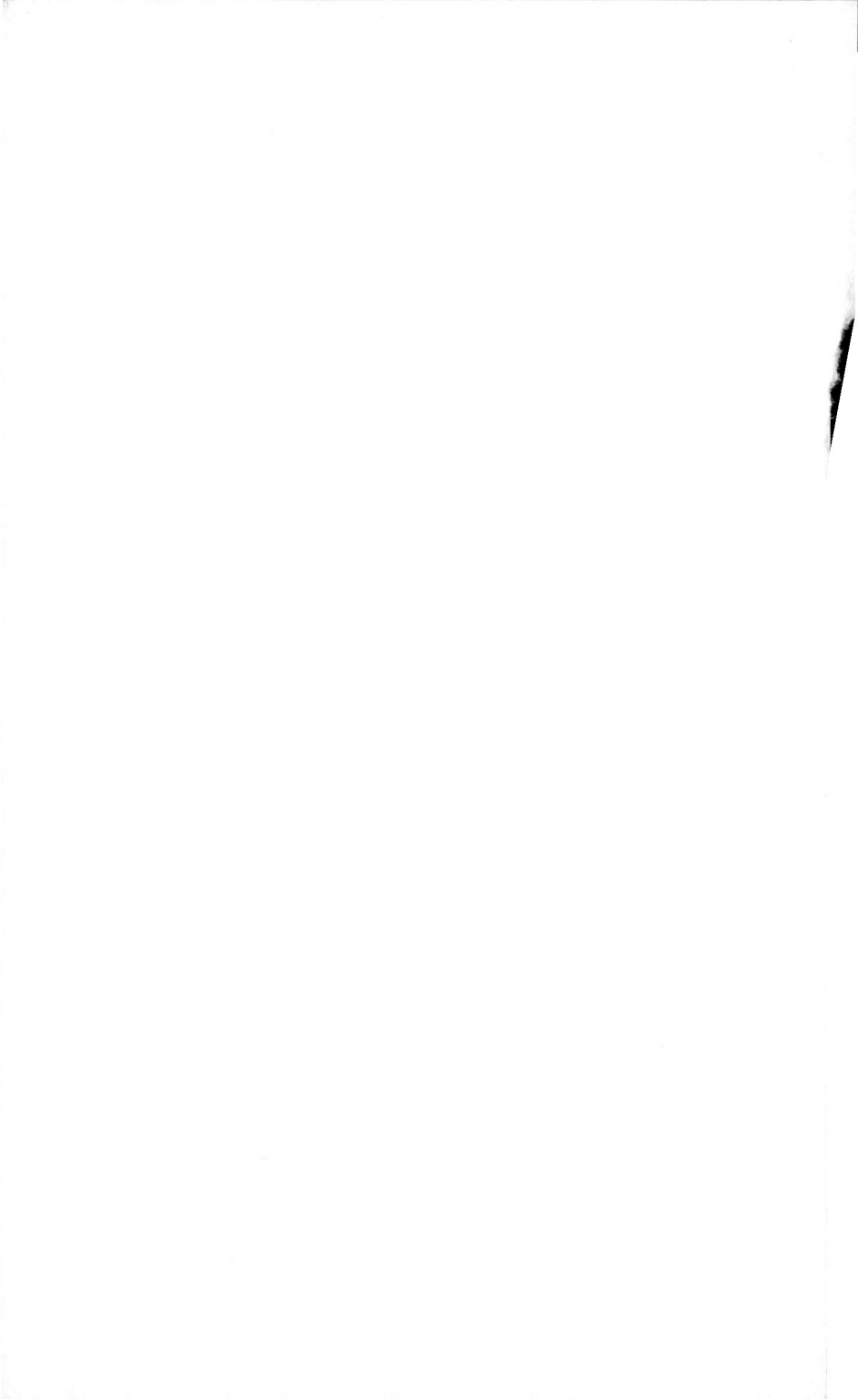